Leading Aerobic Dance-Exercise

SUSAN K. WILMOTH, PhD

HUMAN KINETICS PUBLISHERS, INC.
CHAMPAIGN, ILLINOIS

Library of Congress Cataloging-in-Publication Data

Wilmoth, Susan K., 1955-
  Leading aerobic dance-exercise.

  Bibliography: p.
  Includes index.
  1. Aerobic dancing—Study and teaching.   2. Aerobic
exercises—Study and teaching.   3. Sports medicine.
I. Title.
RA781.15.W55   1986   613.7'1   85-30237
ISBN 0-87322-044-7

Production Director: Ernie Noa
Copyeditor: Olga Murphy
Typesetter: Yvonne Winsor
Text Layout: Denise Mueller
Text Design: Julie Szamocki
Cover Design and Layout: Jack Davis

Cover photo by Jim Corely, courtesy of The Fitness Center in Champaign, Illinois.
Special thanks to Kim Hardin, Fitness Director, and Mary Theesfeld, Sandra Meier,
Debbie Forsten, Steven Jeffries and Bill Sunderland.

Printed by: United Graphics

ISBN 0-87322-044-7

Printed in the United States of America

10 9 8 7 6 5 4 3 2 1

Human Kinetics Publishers, Inc.
Box 5076, Champaign, IL 61820

To

Liz Davis and Mary Hull of The Ohio State University
for giving me the opportunity to teach
aerobic dance-exercise classes

and

Rainer Martens of Human Kinetics Publishers
for giving me a chance

Acknowledgments

When writing a book, there are many people at many different stages of the process to thank for their help. From start to finish I have been blessed with friends and colleagues who selflessly gave me their time to improve my book. At the manuscript stage, I had a team of reviewers whose constructive comments were invaluable. I would like to thank Peg Goyette, Lynn Darby, Roberta Pohlman, Bernie Pignatello, Sally Foster, Marsha Weaver, Melinda Flegel, Gwen Steigelman, Liz Davis, Rainer Martens, and my parents for their excellent suggestions.

I would like to thank my friends at Human Kinetics for their commitment to this project: Olga Murphy for her superb copyediting, Julie Szamocki for her great design, Yvonne Winsor for her excellent typesetting, Ann Bruehler for her fine proofreading, Denise Mueller for her sharp paste-up work, and Ernie Noa, our production director, for his help on the cover design and his continual support throughout the project. Thanks also to Karen Shannon and Dick Flood for their beautiful artwork. And last, but far from least, Tom for his understanding when I needed time to make my dream come true.

Contents

There is something about dancing and music that's magic—it lifts people up. Whether the reason is the music, or the camaraderie, or the behavior-mod technique of encouraging women and men to smile and shout during the workout, [Dance-exercise] has reversed the trend of the lonely, long distance runner.

Time, November 2, 1981 (p. 104)

Preface

Getting a new class started is never easy. Preparing instructors to lead it is even more of a challenge. Five years ago, I suggested getting an aerobic dance-exercise class started at The Ohio State University. As the committee worked its way through the usual steps for implementing a new class, one question was hotly contested: What qualifications did instructors need to teach the class?

While some argued the importance of a strong dance background, others insisted that aerobic dance-exercise was a fitness program and that instructors should be knowledgeable about exercise prescription. It became clear that instructors needed to possess a combination of teaching skills. They needed to have experience teaching dance, prescribing and individualizing fitness programs, and demonstrating leadership skills to attract and to maintain good class attendance. Because I had taught dance and was currently studying exercise physiology, I was selected as an instructor and as a consultant in the instructor selection process. As a consultant, I helped determine what kind of knowledge instructors needed to better prepare them to offer safe programs to their participants.

As our programs were growing at Ohio State, enrollments in programs across the country were also skyrocketing. We discovered that other companies, recreation departments, health spas, and private organizations were also struggling to organize the proper training for instructors. Today, even though 35 different organizations are offering certification programs for aerobic dance-exercise leaders, the question of qualifications is still being examined.

To answer the qualifications question, my own resolution is that each leader should have a basic understanding of exercise physiology, dance-exercise movements, dance-exercise injuries, sports psychology, and leadership skills that contribute to aerobic dance-exercise. The purpose of this book is to help anyone, from any professional background, become the best aerobic-dance exercise leader possible. Whether you are currently leading a class or merely toying with the idea of becoming a leader, the ideas presented here will help you prepare for your classes.

After reading chapter 1, you will be able to assess your current skills and knowledge applicable to aerobic dance-exercise. Once you are aware of what skills you possess, the next step is to work toward overall improvement. Reading reliable fitness information is one way to improve your weaker areas and to enhance your stronger ones. How to select reliable fitness information is also discussed in chapter 1. A list of professional sources from which to obtain reliable aerobic dance-exercise materials is offered in Appendix A.

In chapter 2 you will gain insight into how the body adapts to exercise, which is what aerobic fitness is all about. This chapter begins by familiarizing you with how some of the major body systems function at rest. With this background information, you can more fully appreciate the changes that occur in these systems during aerobic exercise.

Then in chapter 3 you will learn more about how to apply the aerobic information discussed in chapter 2 to your program. You can evaluate the purposes and importance of warming up, working out, and cooling down in each class session. In addition, some basic environmental concerns to consider when designing your class are also discussed.

Books comprised of choreographed aerobic dance-exercise routines fill the trade market book shelves. Although chapter 4 is titled ''Dance Steps and Exercises,'' it was not written to provide you with routines to use in your class. Instead, the purpose of chapter 4 is to help you sharpen your analytical ability to evaluate those dance steps and exercises you choose to include in your routines. You will develop some skills in selecting, leading, and systematically observing the performance of dance steps and exercises. Choreography is briefly discussed in terms of how to match musical energy to exercise energy. How to safely perform exercises as well as what exercises to avoid are also included.

Sports medicine and dance medicine have become closer disciplines because of the need to prevent and to treat aerobic dance-exercise injuries. The prevention and treatment of the most common types of aerobic dance-exercise injuries are discussed in chapter 5. The minor aches and pains a dance-exerciser might experience are also addressed.

Motivating your participants to attend your class regularly will be your constant challenge. In chapter 6 some suggestions are offered on how to determine participants' needs and on how to help them set goals geared toward making exercise a part of their lifestyle. Your own motivation for wanting to be an aerobic dance-exercise leader is also challenged.

Chapter 7, ''Administrative Notes for Aerobic Dance-Exercise Leaders'' deals with such management concerns as legal liability, advertising your program, and salary considerations. Whether you are currently self-employed or are an instructor in a well-established program, you need to be aware of these administrative matters and how they can affect you.

As you are reading, you will note (♪) that many of the chapter titles and major headings are accompanied by song titles. These titles are included not only for your enjoyment but also to reinforce the idea of varying your musical repertoire as you plan for your classes. These tunes cover a variety of musical styles, and you may recognize some of them; but unless your taste in music is quite varied, you will not recognize all of them. The point to be made here is that you will have participants with different musical tastes in your class. A list of these song titles and the names of the albums on which they appear are in Appendix B. Many songs from each of these albums are good ones to use for warming up, working out, or cooling down. Then in Appendix C you will find useful resource materials that will keep you up-to-date on the latest developments in aerobic dance-exercise. For those wishing to study the field more closely, refer to those articles marked with an asterisk (*). These articles represent research-oriented articles on aerobic-dance exercise.

Many of my fondest memories of teaching aerobic dance-exercise at The Ohio State University and elsewhere are of the times when we aerobic dance-exercise leaders gathered together and exchanged ideas. Ideas are a beginning. Open this book with the expectation of finding new ideas, and close it with an appreciation of what it takes to prepare for and to lead aerobic dance-exercise classes. I hope you enjoy your own career as an aerobic dance-exercise leader.

Sue Wilmoth

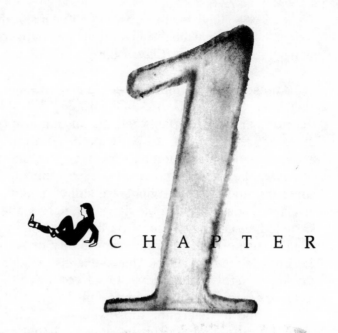

C H A P T E R

The Job of the Aerobic Dance-Exercise Leader

I Hope I Get It

Give me the job and you've instantly got me involved.
Give me the job and the rest of the crowd will get sold.
(From *A Chorus Line*)

An estimated 22 million people are now participating in aerobic dance-exercise programs (Garrick, Gillien, & Whiteside, 1985). This sharp increase in the number of participants reflects an ongoing commitment from more and more dance-exercisers. As participants continue to train they also continue to ask questions concerning all aspects of their training progress. Although a rash of newspaper and magazine articles respond to frequently asked questions, some training misconceptions are still circulating by word of mouth from class to class. Today, the aerobic dance-exercise leader faces a more demanding and knowledge-seeking group of participants than ever before.

Because of the continuing popularity of aerobic dance-exercise, the demand for knowledgeable aerobic dance-exercise leaders is on the rise. But beware, the market is highly competitive. Once you have decided to become an aerobic dance-exercise leader, it is important for you to analyze the skills you currently possess and to determine those you will need to do the job. Rate yourself using the four essential skills in Figure 1.1 that are necessary for being an aerobic dance-exercise leader.

If you are currently leading a class or are preparing to lead one soon, answer the following questions.

- Which is your strongest component as an aerobic dance-exercise leader?
- Which is your weakest component as an aerobic dance-exercise leader?
- Which component needs the most work toward improvement?

Aerobic Fitness Information

Ability to apply this knowledge to your program—low ———————————————— Ability to apply this knowledge to your program—high

Aerobic Dance-Exercise Movements

Knowledge and skills—low ———————————————— Knowledge and skills—high

Preventing Injuries or Providing First-Aid

Knowledge and skills—low ———————————————— Knowledge and skills—high

Leadership Ability

Knowledge and skills—low ———————————————— Knowledge and skills—high

Figure 1.1 Aerobic dance-exercise skill continuums

Mark an X on each continuum to represent your assessment of your present position. Then, if you are currently leading classes, mark an O where you think your students would rate you on each continuum.

Try to evaluate yourself honestly. The harder you work to identify and to improve your weaker areas, the better aerobic dance-exercise leader you will become. As you finish each chapter of this book, turn back to these continuums and reflect upon the ratings you have just made. As you become more familiar with the topics in this book, your ratings should improve.

♪ You as an Aerobic Dance-Exercise Leader
It Might Be You

Most leaders are stronger in some areas and weaker in others. To achieve a high rating on each scale, you would need an extensive background in several subdisciplines of physical education. For example, achieving a high rating on the aerobic fitness continuum requires extensive knowledge in exercise physiology. To rate yourself highly on the dance and movement continuum, you

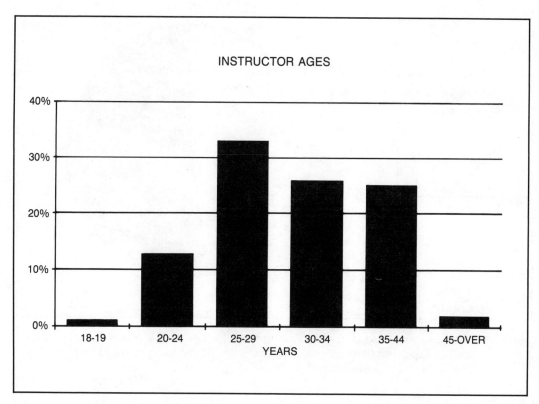

Figure 1.2 Aerobic dance-exercise instructor ages. Note: From *Aerobics & Fitness*, May/June 1985, Vol. **3**, No. 3, (p. 38) by Aerobics and Fitness Association of America. Reprinted with permission.

would need to be well versed in dance and proper exercise selection. The third continuum, which reflects some training in sports medicine, asks you how well prepared you are to prevent and provide first-aid treatment for injuries requiring some training in sports medicine. The last continuum, leadership ability, assesses your knowledge of applying principles from sport psychology to maintain a high level of class attendance and motivation.

Aerobic dance-exercise programs are currently being staffed by leaders of varying ages with diverse professional backgrounds (see Figures 1.2 and 1.3). Amidst this diversity, a common trait surfaces among successful leaders: They capitalize on their strengths and always work toward improving their weak areas. Effective leaders also subscribe to reliable fitness-oriented magazines and materials. They attend workshops and clinics, and continually search for new ideas and information. All of these efforts make their program better and more sound.

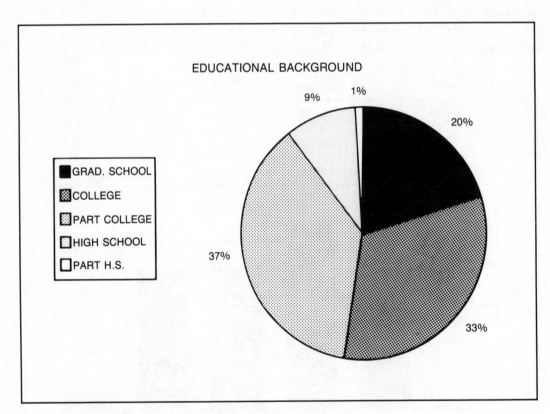

Figure 1.3 The educational background of aerobic dance-exercise instructors. Note: From *Aerobics & Fitness*, May/June 1985, Vol. **3**, No. 3, (p. 38) by Aerobics and Fitness Association of America. Reprinted with permission.

Improving Your Program's Content
I Dowanna' Know

Improving the quality of content of your aerobic dance-exercise program relies heavily on your ability to comprehend and to apply information from the exercise sciences. Selecting reliable information in the area of aerobic dance-exercise fitness can be frustrating and confusing. Add to this the necessity of selecting information in sports medicine and leadership abilities and the task appears overwhelming. The materials available on fitness are plentiful and competitive. However, be careful, for not all information is accurate and reliable. When faced with this abundance of information, exactly how do you go about selecting a reliable source or reference to answer your questions on exercise-related topics?

Credibility is the main concern when evaluating fitness information. Whether exercise topics are discussed in books, magazines, or even on television shows, it's important that you know the credentials of the person(s) presenting the fitness-related information. Become familiar with reputable authorities in the areas in which you are seeking fitness information; otherwise, you may get caught in the celebrity name game.

"What's in a name?" Would it by any other name sell as much? According to the sales figures, books written by celebrities sell quite well. For example, Jane Fonda's *Workout Book* has sold about 1.3 million copies and has been reprinted at least 25 times (Rogers, 1984). Compare that to the 5,000-8,000 copies of books sold, written by such noted exercise physiologists as Jack Wilmore, PhD, and Bud Getchell, PhD. Don't let the popularity of a celebrity influence you. Rather, sort out reliable information from all the information available, and subscribe to those professional journals and magazines that *educate* as well as entertain you. In Appendix A is a list of some sources from which you can begin to compile your aerobic dance-exercise reference materials.

Making Your Program Better
Nature of the Game

Equally important as finding reliable sources of exercise science information is the ability to read and to understand this material. Often, you may not be able to sift through the scientific jargon to understand the practical significance of what is being said. Exercise scientists, like other scientists, seem to speak in their own language. This language enables them to be able to communicate more precisely with each other; however, the specialized terms that make scientific communication easier makes your task of comprehension and application more difficult.

Aerobic dance-exercise leaders need to work hard at bridging the "technical-term gap" between themselves and the exercise scientists. Technical terms from the exercise sciences appear frequently in popular as well as more academic journals. Beyond simply recognizing these popular terms, you need to understand what they mean and how they fit into the overall fitness scheme; therefore, the appropriate technical terms will be used to express the ideas discussed in each of the following chapters. Once you understand the terms and general principles from each chapter, you can then begin to apply them to your program.

 Ease on Down the Road

In chapter 2 some basic concepts from anatomy and physiology are provided as background information to help you better understand how exercise physiologists derive training concepts. Understanding aerobic fitness information and how you can apply it to your program will vastly improve the quality of your program.

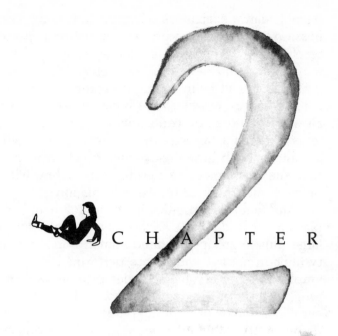

C H A P T E R

Aerobic
Fitness

The Body Shop

Aerobic-dance exercise is a legitimate training method to achieve aerobic fitness. When classes are properly structured, participants will experience many aerobic training benefits. Understanding these benefits will help you to design more sound and individualized aerobic dance-exercise workouts. Many of your participants will be interested in comparing the training benefits achieved from aerobic dance-exercise to the benefits derived from other aerobic activities. However, before you can understand the training adaptations the body systems undergo as a result of exercising (presented in chapter 3), you must first be familiar with how the systems function while the body is at rest. Familiarity with the terminology related to each system will enhance your ability to comprehend authoritative fitness information.

All "aerobic" activities have the following common elements: They (a) place a demand on the cardio (heart) respiratory (lungs) system, (b) use the large muscle groups, (c) predominantly use the aerobic energy system, (d) are rythmic in nature, and (e) are performed at a moderate level of intensity. Examples of other aerobic activities include swimming, walking, jogging, running, and skipping rope. If performed continuously for 20 minutes or more, aerobic activities prompt adaptations (training effects) to occur within the cardiorespiratory, muscular, energy, and nervous systems.

The cardiorespiratory, muscular, energy, and nervous systems adapt to the stress of exercise. Understanding how these systems adapt can help you

- realize the importance of individualized fitness,
- plan safe and beneficial workouts,
- understand training benefits gained from aerobic dance-exercise,
- be better prepared to answer questions concerning exercise, and
- react more logically when confronted with injuries or emergencies.

Before you can understand how a system responds to exercise, you need a basic understanding of how that system functions at rest; otherwise, some of the physiological changes it undergoes may be misinterpreted.

For example, during moderate exercise the heart (cardiovascular system) beats around 150 beats per minute (bpm). This heart rate may sound quite high to someone who does not know that the average resting heart rate is around 68 to 72 bpm. At a moderate level of exercise, the amount of blood being pumped through the heart per minute (cardiac output) increases to 15 liters (1 liter = 1.06 quarts), which is three times the amount of blood being pumped through the body at rest. The demands that exercise places on the systems are much greater than those demands placed on the body at rest.

The body's adaptation to exercise can be studied from the following general levels:

1. Changes that occur at the cellular (biochemical) level—for example, the changes within the muscle cell during different types of exercise. Understand-

ing these responses provides insight about energy production and other chemical processes.

2. Changes that occur in the body's systems—for example, the changes in the cardiorespiratory system such as the amount of blood being pumped per minute to various sites in the body.

3. Other considerations—for example, the influence of environmental factors such as exercising in hot and cold weather and changes in body composition (the amount of fat and of lean weight).

To relate every known or thought-to-happen response to aerobic dance-exercise at each of these levels would take volumes. Your task is to select pieces of information from exercise physiology that are most applicable to designing your program. Not enough information may mean that you will not offer the best program possible or that you will fail to adjust the exercises to each individual's need. Yet, if you tried to learn everything known about exercise, you would not have the time to lead your program. A fair compromise, then, is to become familiar with how the major body systems function at rest as well as during aerobic dance-exercise.

Studying the Body at Rest and During Exercise
If (a Picture Paints a Thousand Words)

The major body systems most involved in aerobic dance-exercise will be examined in the following way: First, how each structure is built and its location in the body will be described; second, how each system functions while the body is at rest will be examined. Then, after you have a basic understanding of how a system works at rest, some changes that it undergoes during the sequential phases (warm-up, workout, and cool-down) of an aerobic dance-exercise class will be discussed in chapter 3. Let's begin with the cardiorespiratory system.

The Cardiorespiratory System
We Go Together

The heart (cardio) and lungs (respiratory) depend upon one another at rest and especially during exercise. Because of this relationship, these two systems are commonly referred to as the cardiorespiratory system. This system receives much public attention because coronary heart disease is so prevalent today. (Aerobic dance-exercise has been associated with a decreased risk of coronary heart disease.) Also, the cardiorespiratory system is now routinely tested to measure an individual's physical fitness level. Let's take a look at the cardiovascular and respiratory systems, respectively.

The Cardiovascular System

With Every Beat of My Heart

The heart weighs approximately 10 oz and is roughly the size of two clenched fists held together. As seen in Figure 2.1, it is slightly left of the center of the thoracic cavity. The heart's interior is divided into four separate compartments, or chambers. The two upper chambers, the *atria* (atrium), and the two lower chambers, the *ventricles*, are connected by valves. One-way valves allow blood to flow from the atria to the ventricles via some of the body's largest blood vessels. Some of these blood vessels carry blood from the heart to the lungs and back to the heart (pulmonary arteries and veins); other blood vessels branching from the aorta leave the heart, supplying blood to the head and neck or the lower body (systemic arteries and veins). The body's blood vessels range in size from a circumference of 1 to 2 inches (i.e., the aorta) to microscopic capillaries. The tiny capillaries weave their way throughout the entire body and are especially numerous in the lungs, skeletal muscles, and skin.

Coronary Arteries

Interestingly, the heart has its own private supply of blood vessels that wrap their way around it (see Figure 2.2). These *coronary* arteries actually sup-

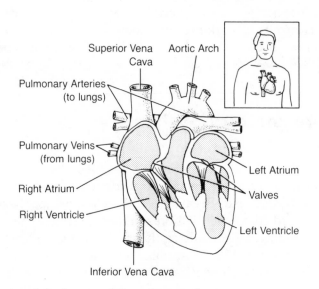

Figure 2.1 The interior of the heart and its major vessels

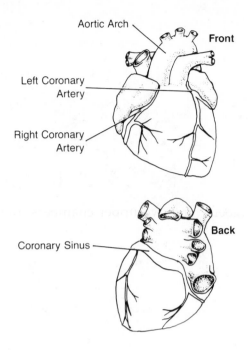

Figure 2.2 The coronary arteries

ply the heart with its nutritional and other needs. Fat deposits may build up in the coronary arteries (as well as in other vessels) and make it difficult for these arteries to supply blood to the heart. If these vessels become completely closed off, the heart is denied its blood supply, and a heart attack will result. While regular participation in aerobic dance-exercise or any other form of aerobic activity provides no guarantee against having a heart attack, it does reduce or help control many of the risk factors that contribute to heart problems.

Cardiac Function

The function of the heart is to pump blood through the body. The pressure of the heart beat forces the blood flow in a continuous, traceable route. This path is shown in Figure 2.3. Blood enters the right atrium, which is a thin-walled storage compartment that receives blood returning to the heart. The blood is forced by atrial contraction through the tricuspid valve into the right ventricle. The ventricles are the heart's pumping chambers and comprise most of the heart's muscle mass. The right ventricle pumps blood through the pulmonary valve into the pulmonary artery and through the lung. After certain gases, mainly oxygen and carbon dioxide, have been exchanged, the blood returns to the left atrium through the pulmonary veins. Left atrial contraction forces blood through the mitral valve into the left ventricle. From the left ventricle blood is pumped through the aortic valve and on through the body.

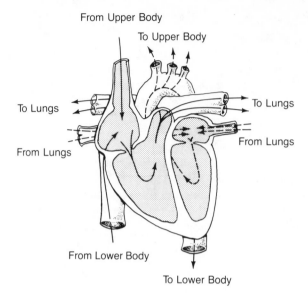

From Upper Body

To Upper Body

To Lungs

To Lungs

From Lungs

From Lungs

From Lower Body

To Lower Body

Figure 2.3 Path of blood flow through the heart

Cardiac Output

The volume (stroke volume) of blood the heart pumps per minute (beats per minute) is referred to as the *cardiac output*. This volume is expressed in liters or milliliters of blood pumped per minute. The symbol $\dot{Q}$ is often used to represent cardiac output in scientific literature or in data tables. Cardiac output is calculated as the stroke volume (the amount of blood pumped out of the left ventricle in one beat) times the heart rate.

$$\dot{Q} = SV \times HR$$

$\dot{Q}$ (liters per minute [l/min]) = SV (liters per minute [l/min]) x HR (beats per minute [bpm])

Your cardiac output changes in proportion to the degree of activity in which you are involved.

The average cardiac output of a person lying down and in a state of complete rest is approximately 5 l/min. Walking would raise the cardiac output to approximately 7.5 l/min. Performing strenuous exercise might cause it to rise to as much as 25 l/min or to around 35 l/min in a highly trained athlete (Guyton, 1974).

There is a maximum rate at which the heart can pump. Within physiological limits, the heart pumps all of the blood that flows into it without excessive damming of the blood in the veins. The amount of blood that the heart can pump each minute depends on two major factors: (a) the pumping effectiveness of the heart and (b) the ease with which blood can flow through the body and return to the heart.

Blood Pressure

If you have ever witnessed someone cutting an artery, even a small one, you'll remember how the blood spurted out. This spurting is an easy way to see how blood under pressure flows throughout the body. As the left ventricle contracts, blood is forced into the systemic arteries, creating pressure. This pressure is transferred to the larger arteries of the body where it can be easily measured. Blood pressure varies from person to person and even within the same person, depending upon the circumstances. For example, your blood pressure is higher when you are standing than when you are sitting, and it is much higher during aerobic exercise than it is at rest.

Despite individual variations, there are normal values for blood pressure. The top number in a blood pressure ratio reading (i.e., 120/80) is the *systolic* pressure. This number represents the blood pressure due to the force of ventricular contraction as it pumps blood out of the heart. The bottom number of the ratio is the *diastolic* pressure and represents the filling of the atria. An average value for normal blood pressure would be 120/80. Mild hypertension ranges between 140/90 to 160/95. High blood pressure, or hypertension, denotes values over 160/95. Regular participation in aerobic exercise has been shown to reduce resting as well as exercising blood pressure.

Redistribution

The body has its own priority system for the amount of blood each of its parts receives. At rest, as seen in Table 2.1, the major organs of the body

Table 2.1 Approximated Shift of Blood From Rest to Exercise

Rest	Exercise
Skin 3-5%	5-10%
Bone 2-5%	.5-1%
Brain 15%	15%
Heart 4-6%	10-15%
Liver Stomach } 30-35% Intestines	3-5%
Kidneys 20-25%	2-3%
Skeletal muscles 15-20%	75-90%

receive the largest amount of blood. During exercise, however, there is a shift of priorities, or redistribution, in some areas to adequately supply blood to the large muscle groups of the arms and legs.

During rest the heart beats approximately 68 to 72 bpm. This value would be lower for anyone who regularly participates in aerobic exercise. Heredity and age are other factors that influence the heart rate: that is, higher aerobic capabilities (i.e., the ability to perform continuous exercise) can be inherited; and as people get older, their aerobic capacity begins to decrease at a rate dependent upon their fitness level.

Individualizing Workouts With a Heart Rate Monitoring System

 You're the One

Each "one" in your class may be at a different level of aerobic fitness. Sometimes you can offer a class and designate the level of instruction (e.g., beginning, intermediate, or advanced). Most likely, you will be confronted with a class of individuals who range widely in cardiorespiratory fitness levels. (Even if you do offer specialized classes according to fitness levels, there is no guarantee that participants have evaluated their own level of fitness accurately.) Your job, then, becomes one of challenging the fit person and, at the same time, pacing the less experienced beginners. Old-timers in advanced fitness categories may be overachievers who push their bodies too far. On the other hand, the cardiorespiratory capabilities of beginners have not been stressed for a long time. To maintain control of the situation, you need to help all participants monitor their heart rate response to your workout so that they do not attempt too much, or too little in trying to achieve the desired training benefits.

In order to handle the increased workload that vigorous physical activity places on the heart, you must slowly begin to train the heart to progressively handle a little more work each time you exercise. This way the heart has plenty of time to adapt to pumping faster and to supplying larger amounts of blood to needed areas. Eventually, you and your heart will be able to perform at an increased workload with ease. This gradual progression in performance and in giving the heart (and lungs) time to adapt to the added stress is what becoming aerobically fit is all about.

Because the heart rate is a reliable and convenient indicator of how much work the cardiorespiratory system is doing during exercise, taking the heart rate has become a routine practice in many aerobic dance-exercise classes. As a leader, you can help individuals measure the amount of work they are doing by periodically having them check their heart rate. It is recommended that heart rates be checked every 7 to 10 minutes during class (Gerson, 1985). This way participants will know whether or not they are working out hard enough to achieve aerobic training benefits. If they are not working out at an adequate intensity, then you need to help them make the necessary adjustments. (Refer to step 4 on p. 18). A good heart rate monitoring system for an aerobic dance-exercise class involves the following steps:

Step 1: Calculating the Heart Rate.

Teach participants to calculate their training heart rate range at the first or second meeting. If you teach this at an orientation meeting, then you can save class time. Prepare handouts of the formula presented here and use posters to reinforce your points.

The following is a commonly used formula (Karvonen's) for calculating a training heart rate for normal, healthy adults along with an explanation of what the numbers represent:

220	A constant value in the formula, representing the heart's anatomical and physiological limits.
minus Age (years)	Remember age, like other factors, influences the heart rate. The maximal heart rate starts to decline progressively at about age 25. The decline is estimated to occur at the rate of 1 beat per year.
minus Resting Heart Rate	Due to individual differences in levels of fitness (as well as other factors), resting heart rates will vary. The best time to take your resting heart rate is the first thing in the morning before getting out of bed. Participants taking medication should check with their physicians concerning possible effects of the medication on resting and exercise heart rates. Some medications commonly used for high blood pressure will lower the heart rate.
multiplied by 60% & 90% (.6) & (.9)	To stress the cardiorespiratory system, you should work out somewhere between 60% to 90% of your maximum heart rate reserve. The American College of Sports Medicine recommends using 60% to 90% of the maximum heart rate reserve (Fox, 1979) for healthy adults.
plus Resting Heart Rate	Due to the variations in participants' resting heart rates, this value is taken into consideration.

**ANSWER:
HEART RATE
TARGET RANGE**

These numbers are your training heart rate range. When performing aerobic activities, par—ticipants should strive to work out within this range for several reasons: This range represents a pace that is sufficient for achieving cardio-respiratory training benefits and that can be easily maintained. For example, if you stay within this range, you should be able to work out for 20 to 30 minutes continually, whereas if you exceed this range, you may fatigue after only 10 to 15 minutes. The lower end of the range is a safe range for beginners, while more advanced participants can work out at the upper end.

For example, to determine a training heart rate range for a beginning level 20-year-old woman who has resting heart rate of 74 bpm, at 60% and 90% maximum you would calculate as follows:

220	(Max HR)	220	(Max HR)
– 20	(Age)	– 20	(Age)
200		200	
– 74	(Resting HR)	– 74	(Resting HR)
126		126	
x .6	(% Max HRR)	x .9	(% Max HRR)
75.6		113.4	
+ 74.00	(Resting HR)	+ 74.00	(Resting HR)
149.60		187.4	

Her exercise training range would be 150-187 bpm.

Step 2: Taking Your Heart Rate.

Teach participants to locate and to count their heart rate. It is easy to find the pulse on the neck (either side of the Adam's apple). Follow your jawline until it ends and press lightly (see Figure 2.4 a). Another convenient location is on the thumbside edge of the wrist (see Figure 2.4 b). Major arteries surface close to the skin at these two sites, creating a strong beat.

Take the count with the index and middle fingers. When taking the pulse on the neck, be sure to apply only light pressure. Excessive pressure may cause the heart rate to slow down momentarily due to a reflexive action.

Have participants practice taking their heart rate a few times prior to the first workout. Establish cue words such as *heart check* to use when it is time for participants to take their heart rate. Insist on quiet during this time to facilitate

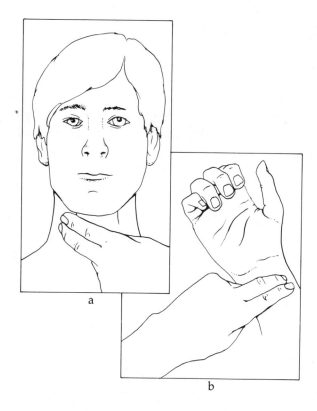

Figure 2.4 Locations for taking the heart rate (a) the carotid pulse (b) the radial pulse

accurate counting, but keep them *moving* rather than standing still. Stopping abruptly can cause blood to pool in the arms and legs and not return to the heart as efficiently as it should. The result can be light-headedness or even fainting. Select another cue word such as *go* and be sure that participants are counting *each* beat after the second you say go until the second you say stop.

To get a minute count, first take a 6-second count and simply add a zero to the number of beats. You can also take a 15-second count and multiply this number by 4. The easiest method is the 6-second count, but the 15-second count is a little more accurate.

Step 3: Benefits of Staying in Your Range.

Explain the benefits and importance of working out within the training range. The benefits are (a) you can be sure of getting just enough of a vigorous workout; (b) you won't fatigue as quickly should you continue to exceed this range; and (c) once you are familiar with working out within this range, you can gauge your participation in *any* aerobic activity.

Step 4: Making Adjustments.

Teach participants how to raise and lower their heart rates by adjusting their performance during class. The heart rate increases when the movements/exercises involve both the upper and lower body. It also increases as the movements are performed in a more exaggerated manner, filling more space. That is, an individual who is working out below (not too common) his or her training heart rate can increase the intensity of the workout by moving the arms as well as by doing the exercises vigorously.

An individual who is working out above his or her training range can do just the opposite—eliminate any unnecessary upper body movements and keep the movements smaller and closer to the body. Similarly, the intensity of locomotor skills, such as jogging, can easily be adjusted to walking.

As participants continue to train, their resting heart rates will begin to decrease 6 to 8 weeks into the program due to adaptations of the cardiorespiratory system. Beginning participants' heart rates will rise high quickly in response to exercise, but as they become more fit, they must work harder at attaining and at maintaining their training heart rate.

Step 5: Visual Aids.

Make posters of the heart rate formula and of locations for taking the heart rate. Include information about adjustments that can be made that affect the heart rate. Skillfully designed posters add color and brighten up the workout area. More importantly, posters help reinforce and remind individuals of the points you've made about working out safely within the training heart rate range.

The Respiratory System
And Every Breath You Take

The lungs are comprised of lobes; the left lung has two lobes and the right lung has three (see Figure 2.5). Inside the lungs is a system of elastic tubes. The largest, the trachea, is about the circumference of a pencil. The trachea divides into bronchi that, in turn, keep branching into smaller tubes. These tubes (bronchioles) continue to branch until they become microscopic air sacs known as alveoli, which are surrounded by capillaries. These alveoli are extremely thin-walled structures that allow a rapid exchange of oxygen (O_2) and carbon dioxide (CO_2).

As you saw in Figure 2.3, the vascular arrangement between the heart and lungs is quite simple. The right ventricle pumps blood into the pulmonary artery. The blood then flows through the pulmonary artery, finally arriving at the pulmonary capillaries that surround the alveoli. After the exchange of gases the

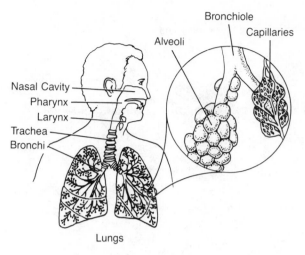

Figure 2.5 The tubular structure of the lungs

blood flows back through the pulmonary veins and eventually back into the left atrium.

The lungs' main function is to aerate the blood. During exercise (as well as during rest), an important exchange is continually occurring between the alveoli and the surrounding capillaries. The major gases being exchanged in greater quantities during exercise are oxygen and carbon dioxide. Oxygen is necessary for energy to be produced, and carbon dioxide is a waste product of this energy production. The exchange is due to the level of concentration of these gases in the alveoli and in the surrounding capillaries. The alveoli have a high concentration of oxygen, whereas the capillaries, because they are carrying blood that has already circulated and delivered oxygen throughout the body, have a high concentration of carbon dioxide (see Figure 2.6). After the exchange of fresh oxygen going into the blood and carbon dioxide going into the lungs to be exhaled, the blood returns to the heart to again be circulated throughout the body. The blood delivers more oxygen to the various sites, whereas the carbon dioxide is blown off with every exhalation.

Aerobic training improves the ability of the heart and lungs to perform this collaborative task of taking in and delivering oxygen to the working muscles during exercise.

How Aerobically Fit are Aerobic Dance-Exercisers?
I Could Have Danced All Night

The term used to represent the quantity of oxygen consumed by the body is *oxygen consumption*. Of the many factors that affect oxygen consumption, the following three are the most important:

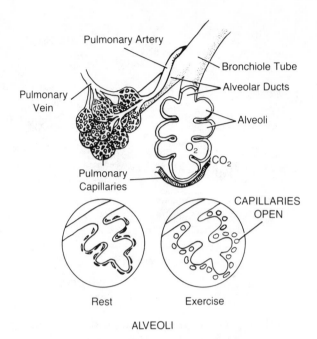

Pulmonary Artery

Bronchiole Tube

Alveolar Ducts

Pulmonary
Vein

Alveoli

O_2

CO_2

Pulmonary
Capillaries

CAPILLARIES
OPEN

Rest

Exercise

ALVEOLI

Figure 2.6 Exchange of carbon dioxide and oxygen between the alveoli and capillaries

1. *Oxygen transport*—the amount of oxygen the blood can carry.
2. *Oxygen delivery*—the amount of oxygen that can get to the active cells.
3. *Oxygen use*—the amount of oxygen that the cells can extract from the blood passing by them.

The amount of oxygen being used per minute by an exerciser is another way (like monitoring the heart rate) of determining the intensity at which a person is working out. Oxygen consumption, or $\dot{V}O_2$, is traditionally measured in liters or milliliters of oxygen consumed per minute (a dot above the V or any symbol denotes a *per minute* measurement). So $\dot{V}O_2$ comparisons can be made among persons of different sizes, $\dot{V}O_2$ measurements are divided by a person's body weight. A $\dot{V}O_2$ measurement therefore is expressed as milliliters per kilogram (1 kg = 2.2 lb) of body weight per minute, or ml/kg/min. The amount of oxygen being consumed at rest (e.g., sitting and reading this book) is approximately 3.5 to 4.5 ml/kg/min. Depending on the pace or intensity of the exercise being performed this resting value can increase to levels of 42.0 ml/kg/min or more.

To determine the intensity of exercise for an individual based on $\dot{V}O_2$, his or her maximal oxygen consumption (max $\dot{V}O_2$) must also be known. Max $\dot{V}O_2$ is the maximal amount of oxygen that you can use per minute. Max $\dot{V}O_2$ is usually determined in a laboratory setting by taking a max stress test. A typical max stress test involves walking, jogging, or running (depending on the individual's level of fitness) on a treadmill under the supervision of a team led by an exercise physiologist. Once a person's max $\dot{V}O_2$ is known then his or her $\dot{V}O_2$ during exercise can be calculated as a percentage of his or her max $\dot{V}O_2$. The American College of Sports Medicine recommends that aerobic exercise be performed at 50-85% of a healthy individual's max $\dot{V}O_2$.

Studies have been conducted to investigate if aerobic dance-exercisers were working out at sufficient intensities as measured by their oxygen consumptions. Weber's (1974) data collected on 10 women reported that aerobic dance required an average of 29 ml/kg/min for 30-minute classes. Foster (1975) studied women ages 20-38 during one aerobic dance routine, and found an average $\dot{V}O_2$ of 33.6 ml/kg/min. These values reflected a high enough percentage of the subject's max $\dot{V}O_2$ to show that participating in aerobic dance-exercise could produce aerobic training effects. As you become more aerobically fit, your max $\dot{V}O_2$ will increase. Rockefeller and Burke (1979) conducted a study with 21 college-age women who were participating in a 10-week aerobic dance class. The class met for 40 minutes, 3 times a week. The average $\dot{V}O_2$ of the women at the beginning of the course was 34.3 ml/kg/min. At the end of the 10th week, their average max $\dot{V}O_2$ had improved to 38.8 ml/kg/min. Vaccaro and Clinton (1981) also noted an increase in their aerobic dance subjects' max $\dot{V}O_2$ from 31.1 to 38.2 ml/kg/min. Vaccaro and Clinton's subjects were college women who participated in 2 hours of aerobic dance a week for 10 weeks.

It is important to be aware that maximal oxygen consumption, like the training heart rate, is also influenced by age, heredity, and level of physical fitness. For example, after the age of 30, there is a slow but progressive loss of lung function. By the age of 65, there may be a decline of approximately 35% in maximal oxygen consumption. Some exercisers have inherited certain physiological characteristics and therefore will have the capability to train to higher degrees of aerobic capacities. The more fit a person becomes, the higher his or her max $\dot{V}O_2$.

A Linear Relationship

To measure the amount of oxygen an exerciser uses per minute is obviously not as convenient as monitoring the heart rate per minute. However, research has shown that the two values increase and decrease as a pair. In other words, when the heart rate goes up, so does the amount of oxygen being consumed. This linear relationship makes many aerobic fitness measurement calculations possible. For example, if you are working at a certain heart rate—even without the elaborate equipment necessary to measure oxygen consumption—it is possible to estimate the amount of oxygen being used. For example, a heart rate of 100 bpm (light work) is accompanied by a $\dot{V}O_2$ of approximately 10 ml/kg/min, whereas a heart rate of 135 (moderate work) denotes a $\dot{V}O_2$ of approximately 20 ml/kg/min (see Figure 2.7).

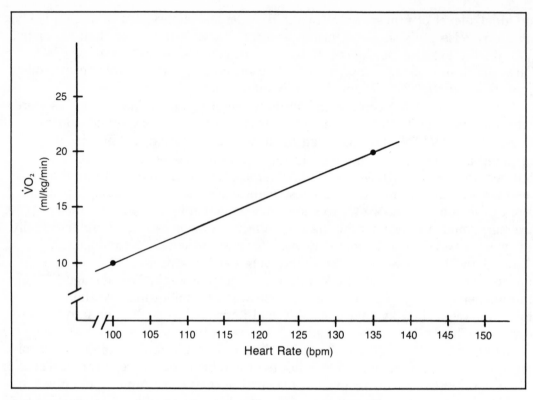

Figure 2.7 The linear relationship between heart rate and oxygen consumption

Caloric Cost

Another interesting physiological relationship is between oxygen consumption and the number of calories expended during exercise. Elementary math has taught us that certain units of measurement can be converted into others: For example, 12 inches equal 1 foot, and 3 teaspoons equal 1 tablespoon. Likewise, the amount of oxygen being consumed during exercise can be converted into the amount of calories being used per minute. For example, when 1 liter of oxygen is used, 5 calories per minute are expended. Hence a 128 pound (58 kg) woman dancing at a moderate heart rate (135 bpm) using approximately 1.16 liters (20/ml/kg) of oxygen would be expending approximately 5.8 kcals (1.16 × 5) a minute. A 154 pound (70 kg) using approximately 1.4 liters of oxygen (20 ml/kg/min) per minute would be expending approximately 7.0 kcals (1.4 × 5) per minute.

This energetic conversion is how exercise physiologists calculate the approximate number of calories being expended during aerobic dance. Most studies tend to agree that by working out at a moderate intensity in your training heart rate range, you will expend between 6 to 8 calories per minute dur-

Table 2.2 Physical Activity and Caloric Expenditure

Work Intensity	Heart Rate	Calories/ min	Activities
Light	Below 120	Under 5	Walking, golf, bowling, volleyball, most forms of work
Moderate*	120 to 150	5 to 10	Jogging, tennis, cycling, hiking, aerobic dance, racquetball, strenuous work, basketball
Heavy	Above 150	Above 10	Running, fast swimming, other brief intense efforts

*Preferred pace for weight control benefits

Note: From *Physiology of Fitness* (p. 88) by Brian Sharkey, 1984, Champaign, IL: Human Kinetics Publishers, Inc. Reprinted with permission.

ing aerobic dance. In Table 2.2 you can compare the caloric cost of aerobic dancing to other activities.

The Muscular System
I Want Muscles

Regardless of how well the cardiorespiratory system might function, movement would not be possible were it not for the muscles and their phenomenal ability to contract. Each muscle has tough, fibrous ends called tendons that attach the muscles to the bones. The middle (belly) of the muscle is thick. If you could cut through the belly of the muscle and look inside, you would see something similar to the cross-section of a muscle depicted in Figure 2.8.

Skeletal muscle is comprised of millions of individual contractile fibers (cells), that are bound together in groups called bundles. Each muscle fiber is wrapped in connective tissue called the endomysium. Just inside and attached to the endomysium is the sarcolemma, or cell membrane. The bundles of fibers are encased in a sheath (perimysium) of connective tissue. This sheath resembles the plastic wrap you use to snugly wrap a piece of meat before you put it in the freezer. Encasing all of the bundles, and hence the whole muscle, is another sheath known as the epimysium. Muscle fibers are richly interwoven with capillaries much like the threads in cloth.

Within these microscopic muscle fibers (cells), contraction, the exchange of oxygen and carbon dioxide with the capillaries, energy production, and many

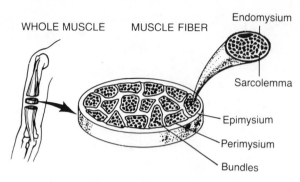

WHOLE MUSCLE   MUSCLE FIBER   Endomysium

Sarcolemma

Epimysium

Perimysium

Bundles

Figure 2.8   Cross-section of a skeletal muscle

other vital functions take place. The fibers' ability to perform these functions is enhanced with regular aerobic activity.

Muscular Fitness

Muscular fitness has three subcomponents: Strength, endurance, and flexibility. Choose and include proper exercises during each class to work on developing all three components.

Muscular strength—the force a muscle or a muscle group can exert during contraction. The result of strength exercises is an increase in the size of the muscle or the muscle group. The enlargement of a muscle group is known as *hypertrophy*. This increase in size results mostly from an increase in size of the muscle fibers themselves. In some animals that have been trained with weights, researchers have noted an increase in the number of fibers comprising the muscle. This observation is yet to be substantiated in humans.

Muscular endurance—the length of time a muscle or a muscle group can continue to exert force without fatiguing. Programs that gradually increase the repetitions (more than 10) of an exercise will also increase muscular endurance. For example, the ability to perform 25 sit-ups demonstrates endurance of the abdominal muscles. You can help participants increase their strength and endurance by including the proper type and number of repetitions of calisthenic exercises during the warm-up and cool-down.

Flexibility—the muscles' increased ability to bend and stretch. Flexibility can be increased by gradual stretching. Most leaders teach flexibility exercises in one of two ways: *statically*—reaching and holding the stretch for about 30 seconds, and *ballistically*—reaching and bouncing for a shorter count of 8 or 10. According to exercise scientists, the preferred method is static stretching. The bouncing movement of ballistic stretching, so often suggested and performed by leaders, can result in a reflexive action of the muscle, causing it to tighten. This, of course, defeats the purpose of getting a nice, slow, full stretch. Bouncing may also cause microscopic tears to occur in the muscle tissue. So please, do not bounce to the beat while stretching. Select music for your stretching exercises that doesn't encourage moving to a beat. Remind your class to relax, to stretch, to hold, to breathe, but *not* to bounce.

Individuals in your class will probably vary greatly in their degree of flexibility. The amount of flexibility at a joint depends upon the joint capsule, the muscle, the tendons, and the ligaments that comprise the joint. Encourage safe (static) stretching practices and individual achievement. Repeat stretching exercises five or six times and hold the final stretching position for 20 or 30 seconds. With the right music, atmosphere, and attitude, participants will find stretching exercises relaxing.

Stretch Break

Teach participants a series of total stretching exercises they can use any time of the day. Doing stretching exercises can be a welcome relief from long hours of sitting and thinking. Good reference books for finding reliable stretching exercises are listed in chapter 7.

Energy Production
Light My Fire

For some, energy is often a rather abstract word. Everyone has it, makes and uses it, but often describes it differently. All of the energy in our solar system originates from the sun, which reaches the earth as sunlight. The millions of green plants that grow on the earth store some of the solar energy as chemical energy and use it to produce their food. Unfortunately, people cannot produce their own food in this manner and must therefore eat plants and animals for their energy supply. Food does not directly supply the energy people need; instead, food is chemically converted into usable nutrients. These nutrients are distributed throughout the body, with some being stored as an energy compound in the body's cells. The energy-rich compound stored within the muscle cells is adenosine triphosphate, commonly referred to as ATP.

The energy the muscles use for contraction is made within the muscle cells. How the energy is made and how fast it is produced depends both upon the type of activity being performed and upon a person's level of physical fitness.

Anaerobic Energy Production

During rest as well as during exercise, as long as ATP is available at the site of the muscle contraction, movement can occur. ATP, however, is available in limited amounts. Because of this limited supply, ATP must continuously be broken down and resynthesized within the muscle cells. Three different energy systems that are capable of resynthesizing ATP have been identified in the body. Two of these systems do not require the presence of oxygen to produce ATP. These quick, energy-producing systems, the ATP-PC and the lactic acid systems are anaerobic systems; they supply energy for short-term, high-intensity exercise. The third system, which works slower and requires oxygen to be present, is the aerobic energy system. Actually, all three systems operate during muscle contraction. The amount of energy needed to sustain an activity and the duration of the activity denotes which system will produce the predominant amount of energy to sustain that activity.

As you begin to work out vigorously there is a temporary shortage of oxygen being delivered to the working muscles. The energy for the first 2 to 3 minutes of the workout is predominantly supplied anaerobically. The skeletal muscles are prepared to produce energy for approximately 2 to 3 minutes without oxygen. But because an aerobic-dance exercise workout lasts for 20 continuous minutes or more, the energy must therefore be predominantly supplied aerobically.

A popular term related to anaerobic energy production you may have heard about is *lactic acid*. Lactic acid is a by-product of anaerobically produced energy. When lactic acid accumulates to high levels in the blood, it causes muscular fatigue. However, the first few minutes of exercise, as well as any change of pace during the workout, would be hindered without the anaerobic energy system and the accompanying lactic acid production.

Lactic acid is not the villain of exercise as it is often made out to be. With training, the body becomes better equipped to deal with lactic acid, because several efficient changes occur (Town, 1985). During training the amount of lactic acid being produced is decreased and the removal of lactic acid from the bloodstream is increased.

Aerobic Energy Production

Aerobic dance-exercise classes usually last for 30 to 60 minutes. All of the dance-exercise steps are performed at a submaximal level of performance, which means that you are working out at an intensity below an all-out, sprinting kind of pace. Because of its submaximal nature, the cardiorespiratory system has plenty of time to deliver the needed oxygen to the working muscles. Thus, the energy for aerobic dance-exercise is predominantly supplied aerobically.

Aerobic dance-exercise at varying intensities (heart rates) and durations (length of the workout) will train the energy systems as well as all the other systems. Training the aerobic energy system requires gradually increasing the amount of time spent doing that activity to give the energy system time to adapt to meeting its new demands.

The Central Nervous System
I Sing the Body Electric

What makes the cardiorespiratory system adjust its activity rate from rest to exercise? What makes the muscles contract and relax at the right time? Somehow, messages must be sent throughout the body to get these systems to speed up and/or to slow down. The main switchboard that organizes these electrical messages is the central nervous system, which is comprised of the brain and the spinal cord (see Figure 2.9). Branching off from the spinal cord and spreading much like the vessels that branch out from the main arteries and veins are millions of various sized nerves. This network of nerves throughout the body allows you to react to your environment.

Let's consider a few things the nervous system does for the cardiorespiratory system and for the muscles at rest and during exercise. Without these lit-

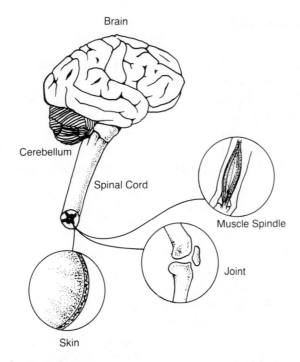

Brain

Cerebellum

Spinal Cord

Muscle Spindle

Joint

Skin

Figure 2.9 The central nervous system

tle electrical signals flowing back and forth between the brain and the various systems, nothing in the body could function.

Signals to the Cardiovascular System

The heart has its own electrical system, much like its private set of coronary arteries (see Figure 2.10). The signals sent over this system are responsible for maintaining a regular heartbeat. Any interference with this electrical network results in an irregular heartbeat, meaning the atria and the ventricles cannot contract in their normal sequence.

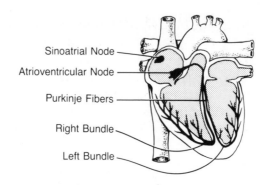

Figure 2.10 The heart's electrical system

A clump of nerve tissue (known as the sinoatrial node), located in the right atrium, receives signals from the brain and sets the pace for the heart to contract. Not surprisingly, this node is often referred to as the heart's pacemaker. The atrioventricular node is located at the junction of the right atrium and right ventricle. The atrioventricular node receives the electrical impulse from the sinoatrial node and sends it to the Purkinje fibers. These fibers, grouped into the right and left bundles, form a network that spreads the impulse throughout the ventricles.

Electrocardiogram

An electrocardiogram (EKG) is a tool used to assess the ability of the heart to transmit its electrical impulses. The EKG mechanically records the heart's electrochemical activity. When the impulse travels through the heart, electrical current generated at the surface of the heart muscle spreads into fluid surrounding the heart. A minute portion of the current flows to the surface of the body (Guyton, 1974). When properly placed on the skin around the heart, electrodes (see Figure 2.10) can pick up this electrical current and transmit it to a recording instrument.

A normal EKG is shown in Figure 2.11. Each segment of the line indicates a portion of the conduction of the heart's current. The curve labeled *P* wave is

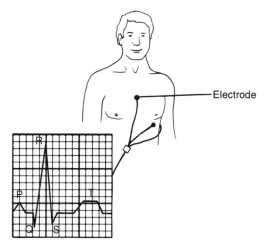

Electrode

Figure 2.11 An electrocardiogram

caused by the current generated as the sinoatrial node initiates an impulse, and the atria contract. The peaks $Q R S$ (the QRS complex) results as the impulse spreads through the Purkinje system, and the ventricles contract. The T wave of the line represents the recovery of the electrical changes in the ventricles. The electrical activity of the ventricles is greater than that of the atria. The weaker atrial recovery is not visible on the EKG.

Taking an EKG is often part of an exercise stress test. Because the heart is performing more work due to the stress of exercise, abnormalities in an EKG are more likely to show up here than during a resting EKG.

The Cardiorespiratory System

Before, during, and after exercise, the nervous system regulates the heart rate. Nervous impulses are also affecting the blood vessels. When necessary, such as during the redistribution of blood from the major internal organs to working limbs in preparation for exercise, the nervous system sends messages to the blood vessels. Vessels supplying certain areas will dilate (become larger) while others will constrict (become smaller).

The rate of breathing during vigorous exercise is also partially controlled by the nervous system. Messages to contract and to help lift the rib cage at a faster rate are sent to the muscles that surround the rib cage.

Signals to the Muscles

Skeletal muscle fibers are united with many nerve fibers. When impulses are sent to the muscles via the central nervous system, they contract, and when the impulses stop, the muscles relax. One motor nerve fiber innervates

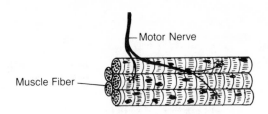

Central Nervous System

Motor Nerve

Muscle Fiber

Figure 2.12 A motor unit

anywhere from 1 to 150 or more muscle fibers. All of the muscle fibers inner-vated by the motor nerve work as a unit: That is, they contract and relax at the same time. Figure 2.12 shows a single motor nerve innervating several muscle fibers.

The nervous system helps to coordinate the functioning of the body's systems at rest and during exercise. Like all other systems, it also responds to training. Its ability to send nervous impulses to the correct site, at the proper speed, and for the necessary amount of time is enhanced through training.

How Sweet It Is

The ability of the body's systems to function together at rest and during exercise is truly amazing. The body's systems are similar to a group of talented musicians orchestrated to play in beautiful harmony. The manner in which these systems respond to exercise has been the focus of a number of research studies. Exercise scientists have identified and described many of the adaptations that occur in these systems as a result of participation in regular, vigorous exercise. A suggested reading list in Appendix C contains recent research articles on aerobic dance.

Because studies have shed light on the training effects of aerobic exercise, some general guidelines have been established concerning the amount, type, intensity, and duration of exercise needed to achieve improvements in fitness. It is essential that as a leader you understand and apply certain training guide-lines/rules when designing your classes.

In the show *Pippin*, King Charlemagne explains the importance of rules to his men by saying, "War is a science with rules to be applied, which good soldiers appreciate, recall and recapitulate, before they go to decimate the other side." Although your intentions are far from decimating the other side, his advice could be rephrased as such: Leading aerobic dance is a science with rules to be applied, which good leaders appreciate, recall, and recapitulate to give their participants the safest, most beneficial workout.

In chapter 3 you will begin to understand how the body systems adapt from rest to exercise. Certain training guidelines that you should consider when designing your classes are covered. Applying these "rules" to all phases of your class will help to individualize the training for all your participants.

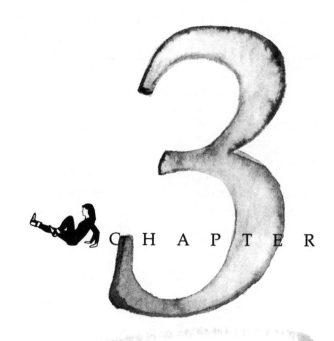

3

Tradition:
Warming Up,
Working Out,
and Cooling
Down

*That's the Way
I've Always Heard
It Should Be*

Traditionally, the format of most aerobic dance classes includes warming up, working out, and cooling down. Although there is nothing wrong with following customary patterns, you need to understand why each phase is necessary. Before deciding to follow any tradition, it is important that you take the time to examine every aspect. A good leader can understand and explain the connection between each phase of class and what is happening in the body's major systems during that phase. This approach to planning class as compared to planning class because "that's the way you've always heard it should be" is much safer.

By further applying the exercise physiology information from chapter 2, you can begin to evaluate the purpose, importance, and proper execution of warming up, working out, and cooling down. You also need to be aware of certain environmental factors that could influence the way in which you conduct class.

Warming Up
Prepare Ye

Preparing the body's systems to make the necessary transitions from rest to exercise is the purpose of warming up. These 3 to 5 minutes of slowly performed, static, overall stretching and light exercises help prepare each system to participate in vigorous exercise. Most exercise physiologists would agree that warming-up is an ounce of injury prevention.

Adjustments

Adjustments are occurring during the warm-up in each of the major systems being stressed during aerobic activities, and these changes can generally be felt. In response to the gradual increase of movement, the cardiorespiratory system begins redistributing blood away from the body's trunk and to the large muscle groups of the arms and legs. Through vasoconstriction (blood vessels becoming smaller) and vasodilation (blood vessels enlarging), more blood is sent to the skeletal muscles of the arms and legs. The nervous system sends signals for an increase in the heart rate, and the lungs begin to increase the rate of breathing. The body's temperature rises by a degree or two, and you begin to sweat. This slight increase in temperature also creates a better environment for the chemical reactions taking place in the muscles to produce energy. The tendons and muscle fibers appreciate the chance to stretch before becoming engaged in vigorous kicking, swinging, and jogging movements.

Guidelines for Warming Up

Make sure everyone in your class warms up with you. Enforce a strict policy of not allowing latecomers to join in after the warm-up is over. The following guidelines will help you plan your warm-up.

LEADING AEROBIC DANCE-EXERCISE

1. Spend the first 3 to 5 minutes of each class warming up. The physiological effects gained from warming up only last for about 15 minutes, so you cannot warm up at 10 a.m. for a 12 p.m. workout.
2. Supervise the warm-up to make sure everyone participates. If everyone warms-up properly many potential aches and pains can be prevented.
3. Perform stretching and calisthenic-type exercises. Stretching exercises will help guard against muscular injury and soreness, while calisthenics will help develop muscular strength and endurance.
4. Establish a routine progression of warm up exercises so that participants will have a sense of structure. For example, you could begin by sitting on the floor, working in a head-to-toe progression of exercises, and then perform a head-to-toe sequence of warm-ups while standing. Keep it interesting by varying the the types of exercises. You can teach 5 to 10 different exercises to stretch out each major muscle group and then vary the ones you lead each class.
5. Plan a well-rounded warm-up for stretching all of the major muscle groups (See Figure 3.1). Select effective, safe warm-ups from reliable books. Be especially careful when selecting warm-up exercises for the neck and lower back. Proper exercise selection is discussed in greater detail in chapter 4.
6. Be prepared to explain the benefits of every exercise you have selected. Participants will often ask what a certain exercise is doing for them as well as ask you to recommend exercises specifically for them.

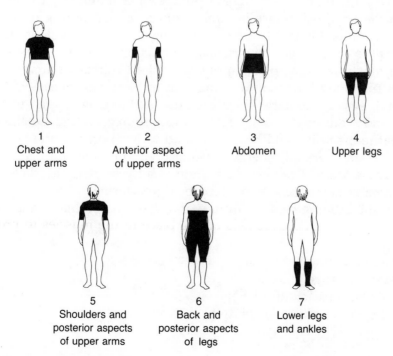

1
Chest and
upper arms

2
Anterior aspect
of upper arms

3
Abdomen

4
Upper legs

5
Shoulders and
posterior aspects
of upper arms

6
Back and
posterior aspects
of legs

7
Lower legs
and ankles

Figure 3.1 The major muscle groups

7. Suggest that warm-up time is a good time to relax the mind. Cheerfully tell participants to forget their cares for the next hour and to concentrate on the good they are doing for their bodies.
8. Always consider the temperature when planning and leading class. Extremely hot and cold days can place additional physiological demands on the body.

The Workout
Let Them Work It Out

After a thorough warm-up, you are ready to progressively pick up the pace and get into a vigorous workout. How the time is spent during this phase of class will determine the extent of the training benefits participants will achieve.

As the workout begins, both the heart rate and number of breaths per minute will increase rapidly. This marked increase is necessary to begin making adjustments in the cardiorespiratory system to adapt to exercise. After a minute or so, both rates will tend to level off to a slower but steadier pace (steady-state). This is important to remember as a leader because monitoring the heart rate after the first song of the workout could be misleading: The higher heart rate would give a false indication for gauging the rest of the workout. Wait at least 4 or 5 minutes into the workout before taking heart rate checks.

Along with an increase in heart rate, there is also an increase in the volume of blood (stroke volume) being pumped per minute by the left ventricle. The reason for this increase in stroke volume is that during rest, only about half of the total amount of blood refilling the left ventricle is pumped out per beat. Due to the stronger ventricular contractions demanded by exercise, however, a much more complete emptying of the ventricle occurs.

Most of the blood flow is now being sent to the major muscle groups of the arms and legs. The muscle fibers are busy exchanging oxygen with the capillaries, and the lungs are busy taking in more oxygen and exhaling carbon dioxide. As the breathing and heart rate tend to level off and the body goes into a steady-state workout, energy is being predominantly supplied by the aerobic energy system. The nervous system is busy helping the skeletal muscles coordinate the exercises-dance steps being performed.

Some of the training benefits from working out aerobically on a regular basis are

* a decrease in resting heart rate,
* an increase in stroke volume,
* an increase in cardiac output,
* an increase in the muscle's ability to extract oxygen,

- an increase in the volume of blood in the cardiovascular system,
- a decrease in resting blood pressure, and
- an increase in the overall efficiency of the cardiorespiratory system.

Too Much, Too Little, Just Right

Three important guidelines to follow when designing the workout in terms of individual fitness are meeting the proper *intensity*, *duration*, and *frequency*. These three factors will influence the extent of the training benefits that participants achieve and will serve as guides to improve their levels of fitness.

Intensity—refers to "how much" exercise each participant is doing during the workout. The intensity of the workout can be gauged by monitoring the heart rate as explained in chapter 2. When working out below the training heart rate range, you are not placing enough of a demand on the cardiorespiratory system to achieve much of a training benefit. Conversely, when working out above this rate, you may fatigue sooner than necessary. Thus, you will not be able to sustain the workout as long, and you will fail to place the continuous stress on the cardiorespiratory system that is desired.

The intensity of a workout can also be gauged by how a participant feels while working out. Dr. Gunnar Borg, a Swedish psychologist, developed what he called perceived exertion ratings. His studies showed that a person's subjective estimate of his or her exercise effort was highly related to that person's heart rate, oxygen consumption, lactic acid levels, and other physiological responses monitored during the workout. In other words, if a person feels as if the workout is too intense, it probably is. In Table 3.1 you can see how his subjective ratings match up against the physiological ones.

An individual who is unfit or who is at a low level of fitness, will reach his or her training range quickly and perhaps even exceed it during the workout. On the other hand, a more physically fit person may have to do more vigorous movements during the workout to reach his or her training range. Proper intensity for the workout, then, is to stay within the established heart rate range as discussed in chapter 2. This in turn will have a positive effect on the next variable of training—duration.

Duration—refers to "how long" each workout should last. Exercise scientists say that to maintain a reasonably fit cardiorespiratory system, an individual should be able to sustain a vigorous workout for 20 to 30 minutes. However, a beginner obviously cannot be expected to work out for 20 minutes nonstop during his or her first class. The goal of 20 to 30 minutes must gradually be achieved over a period of 8 to 12 weeks. During this time, the duration of the workout is increased in reasonably progressive increments.

Beginners need to increase the length of their workout gradually. A safe goal would be to have them work toward adding 2 to 3 routines per week to

Table 3.1 Perceived Exertion

How Does the Exercise Feel?	Rating[a]
	6
Very, very light	7
	8
Very light	9
	10
Fairly light	11
	12
Somewhat hard	13
	14
Hard	15
	16
Very hard	17
	18
Very, very hard	19
	20

[a]The rating multiplied by 10 is approximately equal to the heart rate. For example, ''Fairly light'' = 11 × 10 = a heart rate of 110.

Note: From ''Perceived exertion: A note on history and methods'' by G. Borg, 1973, *Medicine and Science in Sports*, **5**, pp. 90-93. Reprinted with permission.

their workout. Beginners need to be taught to ''listen'' to their bodies for signs of how the body is responding to the additional workload. The body has a remarkable ability to signal a person when he or she is overtraining. Some common warning signals would include the following:

• Nausea after working out
• Shortness of breath (lasting for more than 10 minutes after exercising)
• Prolonged fatigue (even after 24 hours)
• Dizziness
• Light headedness/fainting
• Severe pain in the chest or arms
• Loss of coordination
• Sudden loss of vision
• Confusion
• Fluttering of the heart

If any participant experiences one of these symptoms and the symptom does not go away after exercise is stopped, he or she should seek medical assistance immediately.

Frequency—the number of workouts per week. Working out three times a week is the frequency generally recommended for individuals who desire to maintain some ''cardioprotection'' level of fitness. A beginner who is attempting to establish an aerobic base may often work out 4 days in a row. This format establishes discipline, permits the same level of workout to be done on a regular basis, and can motivate a person to do some serious training. Once an individual has progressed to comfortably working out for 20 minutes nonstop at his or her training heart rate, three times a week will suffice.

Individuals who wish to keep increasing the duration of the workout time beyond 20 minutes should increase the time in small increments just as they did when slowly progressing to the point of a continuous 20-minute workout. They should also pay close attention to their bodies for warning signals of overtraining. Overtraining often brings more problems (injuries, mental anguish,etc.) than it does benefits.

Another way to increase cardiorespiratory fitness is to supplement dance-day workouts with other forms of aerobic activities such as jogging, bicycling, or swimming. As a leader, remind participants that although they can sustain a 20-minute aerobic dance-exercise workout comfortably, they still need to start slowly with their new activity and gradually build up to a 20-minute workout. An aerobic dancer-exerciser's heart and lungs may survive plunging into a 20-minute jog, but you can bet the muscles won't stop complaining for several days!

Doing the Best That You Can Do

As a leader, it is your responsibility to closely examine your teaching situation and to determine how these training factors (intensity, duration, and frequency) have been applied. Perhaps you will join a staff or take a position in which the structure of the workout has already been decided. The schedule, determined months in advance, has aerobic dance-exercise classes meeting on Tuesdays and Thursdays from 6:15 to 6:35. Your first task is to find out why these classes are not meeting three times a week and for more than 20 minutes each time. After all, your class will need an adequate amount of time to warm up, to work out, and to cool down. Talk to the person in charge of scheduling classes. Present your reasons for requesting changes and be prepared to hear some old excuses such as, ''It's a class offered for women only, and the men's basketball program is well established and needs the gym every other evening,'' ''These are the nights the participants themselves chose,'' ''The previous leader set up the class this way, and we assumed she knew what she was doing,'' and ''We didn't know that a certain frequency and duration were needed for aerobic workouts.''

If you can't change the class schedule this time, perhaps you can convince the person in charge of scheduling to plan on changes in the future. (If this seems unlikely to happen, you may wish to find another job). Meanwhile, you face the challenge of educating your class about the need for working out three times a week to achieve aerobic benefits. This can be accomplished in several ways (e.g., minilectures and posters), which will be discussed more thoroughly in later chapters.

Guidelines for Working Out

To plan your workout, use the following important guidelines:

1. Use the proper intensity, frequency, and duration with respect to the fitness level of the participants.
2. Have beginners work out for short periods of time at the lower limit of their training heart rates, and then gradually lead them into longer, more vigorous workouts.
3. Encourage the more fit participants to give it all they've got during the workout and yet to stay within their training heart rate range.
4. Memorize the adjustments that can be made to help individuals increase or decrease their training heart rate (see p. 18).
5. Plan a workout that not only elevates the heart rate but that also uses the major muscle groups of the body continuously.
6. Evaluate your teaching situation ahead of time to incorporate possible changes or to compensate for the conditions with which you are faced.
7. Sharpen your observation skills. If an individual is going to have problems such as injury or dizziness, it will most likely happen during the workout. You will want to be prepared. (Chapter 4 will help you become a good systematic observer.)
8. It's so easy for everyone, *especially the leader*, to get caught up in a fast-moving, popular song, and thus work out at levels way beyond the training heart rate range. Occasionally remind everyone of this, and always be attentive to signs of distress.

Cooling Down
Take It Easy

Spirits high, pulses low is an ideal description of how participants should feel during the last song of the cool-down and as they leave your class. Everyone should feel a sense of satisfaction from the workout (spirits high) and be physiologically recovered from it (pulses low—below 100 bpm).

At the end of the workout, the body's systems must have time to gradually return to their resting states. Every change that occurred as a result of warming up and working out must reverse itself. For example, the redistribution of the blood slowly shifts back from the large amounts in the working muscles of the arms and legs to the original resting sites. This shift takes place more effectively if the intensity of the exercise is reduced gradually rather than halted abruptly. Plan an *active* cool-down. Have participants keep moving at low intensities so the muscles of the arms and legs continue to contract, for these contractions act as pumps to help the blood return to the heart. As the intensity of the workout tapers off, the breathing rate will slowly return to resting values. The muscles are ready for easy, slow stretches to assist the recovery from vigorous movements. The nervous system is busy sending signals to reroute the blood, to slow down the heart rate, and to get the muscles to slow down their production of energy in preparation to return to their resting state.

The cool-down should include walking and slow overall stretching exercises. The cool-down should last for 10 to 15 minutes or *until* an individual's heart rate recovers to below 100 bpm.

Relaxation Techniques

The cool-down period is an ideal time to lead some relaxation exercises. Like fitness training, relaxation training requires regular practice to yield results. If you want to include relaxation techniques as part of your cool-down activities, set aside at least 10 to 15 minutes at the end of the session for doing them.

Progressive relaxation training was developed by Edmund Jacobson in the 1930s. Recently, this type of training has been modified by psychologists, sport psychologists, and others to make the procedures easier to teach and more effective for the participants. The purpose of relaxation training is to have participants recognize their tense feelings and work toward replacing those feelings with more relaxing ones. The procedure consists of having participants alternately tense and then relax the major muscle groups in a sequential manner. The following is a workable sequence of muscle groups:

> Right toes/left toes
> Right foot/left foot
> Right leg below the knee/left leg below the knee
> Right leg below the hip/left leg below the hip
> Both legs below the hip
> Stomach muscles/buttocks
> Right fingers/left fingers
> Right arm below the elbow/left arm below the elbow
> Right arm below the shoulder/left arm below the shoulder
> Chest muscles
> Neck muscles
> Jaw muscles
> Forehead
> Entire face and head
> Entire body

To teach this technique, have participants assume a comfortable lying or sitting position on the floor with their eyes closed. Have participants tense the specific area of the body, hold for about 20 seconds, and then relax. Repeat with the next muscle group and so on until you have covered all of the muscle groups. Speak calmly, telling participants to feel the tension as they are holding and to feel the tension leaving as they are relaxing.

Guidelines for Cooling Down

To cool-down, use the following guidelines:

1. The cool-down should last approximately 10 to 15 minutes.
2. Gradually taper the intensity level of the routines.
3. Use an active cool-down involving light-intensity exercises and stretching.
4. Begin with a few standing cool-down routines before doing routines sitting or laying on the floor.
5. Be sure that everyone's heart rate recovers to below 100 bpm before leaving class.
6. Incorporate some relaxation exercises that individuals can perform on their own.
7. Enforce a policy of not allowing anyone to leave class before sufficiently cooling down.

Suggested outlines for structuring classes for all levels are presented in Tables 3.2, 3.3, and 3.4.

Table 3.2 Sample Beginner's Class

Duration/ Minutes	Type of Exercise	Music
3-5	Sitting upper body flexibility	Slow
3-5	Sitting lower body stretching	Slow
3-5	Side lying stretches and sit-ups	Slow
3-5	Standing stretches for upper and lower body	Moderate
10-15	Aerobic dance-exercise workout (Use combination fast-walking and slow-jogging moves)	Fast
3-5	Taper down using slow-moving exercises while standing	Moderate
3-5	Cool-down using stretches and relaxation exercises	Slow

Environmental Concerns

Stormy Weather

In terms of exercise, stormy weather can be a hot, humid day or a cold, blustery one. Take temperature into account when planning classes for summer

Table 3.3 Sample Intermediate Class

Duration/ Minutes	Type of Exercise	Music
3-5	Sitting upper body flexibility	Slow
3-5	Sitting lower body stretching	Slow
3-5	Side lying stretches and sit-ups	Slow
3-5	Standing stretches for upper and lower body	Moderate
15-20	Aerobic dance-exercise workout	Fast
3-5	Taper down using slow-moving exercises while standing	Moderate
3-5	Cool-down using stretches and relaxation exercises	Slow

Table 3.4 Sample Advanced Class

Duration/ Minutes	Type of Exercise	Music
3-5	Sitting upper body flexibility	Slow
3-5	Sitting lower body stretching	Slow
3-5	Side lying stretches and sit-ups	Slow
3-5	Standing stretches for upper and lower body	Moderate
20-35	Aerobic dance-exercise workout	Fast
3-5	Taper down using slow-moving exercises while standing	Moderate
3-5	Cool-down using stretches and relaxation exercises	Slow

and winter; otherwise, serious problems may result. A good leader is prepared to make adjustments in leading the class as the temperature dictates.

Working Out In a Heat Wave

Two major problems, dehydration and heat illness, can occur when vigorously working out in a hot (temperature exceeding 85° F) or humid (humidity above 85%) environment. Dehydration is a loss of water due to heavy sweating; heat illness is due to overheating. Because most aerobic dance-exercise classes are held indoors, these problems are reduced; however, they should still be taken into account, for the room may not be properly air-conditioned.

The body has a fairly good heat-regulating system that controls the body's ability to maintain a stable body temperature of 98.6° F. This regulating system responds to the temperature of the blood as it flows by a special area in the brain. When the blood is warmer than it should be, the nervous system signals for more blood to be routed to the skin and to activate the sweat glands. When this happens, heat is lost by conduction, a transfer of heat between different temperatures in direct contact with each other. When the air temperature is cooler than the skin, the heat is drawn away from the body. (The additional blood being sent to the skin increases the workload of the cardiovascular system).

If the heat load is still too much for the body to handle, the sweat glands are activated during exercise. Water is released from the body in another attempt to aid in this heat loss. However, the body is only cooled if the sweat evaporates. If the sweat cannot evaporate, or change into vapor, due to high humidity, no cooling can take place because the air is already heavily saturated with water.

It is crucial that leaders recognize signs of heat illness. Equally important, the leader must educate the participants through a minilecture or some means about the symptoms of heat illness and know and teach the proper first aid treatment for each symptom. Summarized in Table 3.5 are the stages of heat illness, accompanied by the proper first-aid treatment.

Table 3.5 Heat Illness Symptoms and First Aid

Stage	Symptoms	First Aid
Heat Asthenia	Fatigue, headache, heavy sweating, high pulse rate, poor appetite, insomnia.	Move to a cooler, dryer place. Drink plenty of fluids. Rest.
Heat Cramps	Painful muscle spasms, pupils dilate with each spasm, skin cool and clammy.	Apply firm pressure on cramping muscles.
Heat Exhaustion	Profuse sweating, weakness, vertigo, skin cold and pale, possible vomiting.	Move to cooler area immediately. Bed rest. Seek medical help.
Heat Stroke	Weakness, vertigo, sweating stops just before heat stroke, nausea.	Severe medical emergency. Get a doctor.

Some ways to prevent heat illness are by (a) replacing water frequently, (b) dressing properly, and (c) adjusting or cancelling class if necessary.

Water replacement—explain to your participants the importance of drinking water before, during, and especially after exercising. Encourage individuals to drink water at any time during the workout, but caution them to drink only small amounts of water (3 to 6 oz). Otherwise, they may tend to feel uncomfortable.

Proper clothing—when exercising in the heat, wear lightweight and loose-fitting clothes. The more absorbent materials such as cotton are preferred because they help body heat to escape. Rubberized sweat suits or anything that will increase sweating, yet acts as a barrier to prevent heat loss, can cause the body to overheat. Enforce a strict policy on dressing appropriately to workout in the heat, and this will be one less contributing factor to heat illness.

Cancelling the class—don't let participants persuade you to hold class against your better judgement. Rather consider the following factors in determining cancellation: First, consider the *time* of day the class is to be held. If you can hold class earlier in the morning or in the evening, do so; but if your class meets at noon, proceed with caution. Second, consider the *temperature* and *humidity*. If they both are high and the class is to be held at noon, you have twice the problems. Third, consider the *fitness level* of those you are leading. The more highly fit individuals will be able to handle the added stress of heat much better than will the less fit.

Guidelines for Hot Weather Workouts

Use these guidelines when planning to work out in hot weather.

1. Hold summer classes in the early morning or evening hours.
2. Encourage participants to drink water whenever they need it, especially before and after class.
3. Check heart rates periodically. Explain to the class that their heart rates will reach their training zones more quickly due to the heat. Encourage everyone to stay within his or her heart rate zone.
4. Memorize the symptoms associated with dehydration and heat illness: headache, nausea, weakness, and the more severe symptoms of cessation of sweating, confusion, and collapse.
5. *Plan Ahead*. Establish good emergency procedures in case an individual suffers from heat illness. Have preplanned answers to such questions as, Who takes care of that person? If the leader is responsible, then who is in charge of conducting class, or is class over? What first aid plans do you have? Where can you get medical help if you need it?
6. If necessary, exert your authority as the leader and cancel a class instead of leading an unsafe workout.

Cool Weather Workouts

Leading a class during cold weather doesn't present nearly as many problems as working out in the heat. However, the leader needs to be aware of a few things.

Exposure to the cold causes the blood vessels to constrict, thereby reducing the amount of blood flowing to the arms and legs. This occurs to help the body conserve heat (unlike trying to lose it in hot weather). Because many participants will have just come in from the cold and the room itself may be a little cool, the warm-up period during cold weather should be a little longer. The body needs time to adjust to increasing the circulation to the arms and legs.

Also important is that the participants are sufficiently cooled down and properly dressed before going outside into the cold. Damp clothing conducts heat away from the body, so a change of clothing or extra layers to wear over the damp clothes are recommended. Because much of the body's heat escapes through the hands and head, you might suggest that they wear gloves and hats as well.

Guidelines for Cold Weather Workouts

Use the following guidelines for planning classes during the winter:

1. Lengthen the amount of time spent in warming up. Cold muscles are more susceptible to injury.
2. Lead an active cool down making sure participants do not go outside overheated.
3. Dress appropriately for class and before going back outside after the workout.

 We've Only Just Begun

The more you utilize the information from exercise physiology in your class—whether it be in the planning stages, actually leading the class, or by other educational visual aids such as posters—the better quality program you will have. These first three chapters have merely highlighted some information from exercise physiology to help you plan and lead your class more effectively. These chapters are just a beginning, and this book is only the start of your learning process. Much more aerobic fitness information is available, so you must make an effort to stay up-to-date with the current trends. Some resource materials that will keep you up-to-date on the latest fitness information are listed in Appendix A.

Once you've established a workable scientific base from which to lead, it's time to move on to other aspects of leading. Various dance-exercises and teaching styles that you may want to use in leading your class are examined closely in chapter 4.

Dance Steps
and Exercises

Best That You Can Do

Throughout your aerobic dance-exercise days, you have probably performed quite a few dance steps and exercises. As the leader, you need to feel confident that each dance step and exercise in your repertoire is safe and beneficial. Knowing how to select, to lead, and to systematically observe dance-exercises helps you to develop a safe and purposeful program. Therefore, the purpose of this chapter is not to present aerobic dance-exercise routines or exercises to include in your program, but to help you develop some skills in the areas of selecting, leading, and systematically observing dance steps and exercises. These skills will help you evaluate all kinds of aerobic dance steps and exercises you may already be doing in your class or are planning to include in the future. Some general features of selecting, leading, and systematically observing apply to both dance steps and exercises. Other aspects only apply to dance or exercises.

General Considerations
Both Sides Now

When selecting aerobic dance steps and exercises to present to your participants, you need to ask, "What is this step/exercise doing for the participant?" For each step/exercise, you should be able to answer the following questions:

1. *The purpose:* Will performing this step/exercise increase strength? Flexibility? Cardiorespiratory fitness?
2. *The proper execution:* What is the safe way to perform this step/exercise from beginning to end?
3. *Common errors:* What are some common errors participants *could* make while performing this step/exercise that, if not corrected, will either reduce the benefit or possibly do more harm than good?
4. *Number of exercises:* How many steps/exercises will need to be performed on each side of the body to achieve the desired purpose or training effect?
5. *Name:* What name will you give the step/exercise so that the class can identify it from routine to routine?
6. *Variations:* What are some safe variations of this step/exercise, that could add variety to the workout?

Organizing this information on a file card makes it readily available and, if applicable, easy to share with other leaders in the program. A sample file card would look like this:

Name: Push-up.

Purpose: To develop strength and endurance of the back of the arms, chest, and shoulder muscles.

Proper execution: Spread the feet 2 to 4 in. apart; relax the knees; do not lock them. Hold up the buttocks a little bit above the line of the rest of the body. (This will protect the lower back.) Hold in stomach muscles; do not let them sag. Spread apart fingers. No undue strain should be felt in the wrists. Do not lock the elbows when your arms are fully extended, nor overbend them at the lowest portion of the push-up. Keep the head aligned with the body throughout the exercise.

Common errors: Keeping buttocks in alignment with the rest of the body, locking elbows during full extension, not tightening the abdominal muscles, and holding the breath while performing the exercise.

Repetitions: Depending upon fitness level of your class, suggested progression would be 5 reps for beginning levels, 10 to 15 reps for intermediates, and 15 to 25 reps for advanced levels.

Variations: Have participants shout out one of their favorite fattening foods on the way down and a healthy substitute on the way up.

Once you have carefully selected the dance steps/exercises you are going to use, the next step is planning how to lead the class using them.

Leading and Demonstrating Dance Steps and Exercise
Follow Me

When leading the class you perform a dual role: (a) you are vocally calling out cues for the class, and (b) you are demonstrating the exercise at the same time. Some participants will catch on to the exercise more quickly by watching you, while others will appreciate your vocal cues. The ideal situation is, of course, to perfectly coordinate what you say to what you do. Nothing will lessen your credibility faster than instructing the class to perform an exercise one way while you perform it incorrectly another way.

Vocal Cues

Calling out the name of the next exercise-dance step to be done, or more importantly, key point reminders for performing the exercise properly (i.e.,

"Let's hold and not bounce") are examples of vocal cues. When preparing to go to the next exercise-dance step, make a smooth transition by phrasing your cue to the count of the music. Also, call out the next exercise in advance, as a square dance caller would. For example, you are working out to a song in 4/4 time, and all of your exercises-dance steps consist mainly of sets of 4 (i.e., 4 jumping jacks followed by boogie steps with knee lifts and then repeat the phrase). Prepare the class to change exercises by saying, "Let's (count 1) Change (count 2) To (count 3) Boogies (count 4) On (count 1) The (count 2) Next (count 3) Beat (count 4). This way everyone keeps moving, knows what's coming next, and can change direction quickly without colliding into anyone else.

Demonstrating the Exercise

The main considerations in demonstrating an exercise are to perform it correctly and simultaneously with the vocal cues. It is also a helpful habit to use your hands to lead the class, much like a symphony conductor leads musicians. Appropriate, well-timed hand gestures can prevent you from becoming hoarse from shouting over the music for an hour. Hand motions can indicate a change of direction, change of speed, or an increase in the intensity of movement. Hand motions can also be used to make a movement look more graceful, to assist in fluid transitions, and to clap your approval of the class's performance.

Each exercise and dance step you intend to teach participants must be demonstrated effectively and performed proficiently. If you are not certain about your ability to perform a particular exercise-dance step, either practice it until you can perform it effectively or seriously consider leaving it out of the routine.

The four stages of presenting an effective demonstration (Martens, Christina, Harvey, & Sharkey, 1981) that you can apply to leading aerobic dance are outlined as follows.

Stage 1: Prepare the participants for the demonstration—to teach any exercise-dance step effectively, first get the participants' attention. Some attention-getting devices are to turn the music down or off or and to wait until after a fast routine when most participants become quiet. It's important to maintain a balance between teaching new exercises-dance steps and keeping participants moving. In a beginners's class, the problem is easily solved by interspersing new exercises-dance steps between routines. This gives the heart rate time to recover and also provides for an active (everyone moving) recovery. In an intermediate or advanced class, teach new exercise/steps after the warm-ups or as part of the cool-down period.

Stage 2: Demonstrate and explain the new exercise-dance step—to start, face the class and demonstrate and explain the new exercise-dance step. Give clear, concise explanations and perform the entire movement. Then repeat the exercise-dance step again but at a slower pace. When participants are ready to try it, turn around and do the exercise-dance step with your back to the class; this way they can follow you precisely and not have to do it backward as they would be if you were still facing them.

During the demonstration be sure and call their attention to any common errors that could occur while performing the move. Demonstrate the exercise-dance step first without music and then once with it. If you yourself have practiced demonstrating and explaining the step or exercise, teaching it to participants can be done quickly and effectively.

Stage 3: Name the new exercise or step—give the new exercise/step a name; then each time you call out this name during the routine, everyone will be able to follow you and to keep on moving. Once participants are familiar with the name, you can use the exercise/step in new routines, without having to stop and go over it.

Stage 4: Answer relevant questions about the new exercise/step—after you have given the demonstration, ask participants if they have any questions. Some participants might ask you to repeat the demonstration several times until they are comfortable performing it. Rather than give repeat performances, however, assure these participants that the new exercise/step will be used throughout the routine and that by the end of the class they will have it grasped it. Further, make yourself available before and after class for anyone who has questions on how to perform any of the exercises-dance steps.

Systematic Observation

Private Eyes (Are Watching You)

As you are leading, both verbally and nonverbally, it is your responsibility to keep a sharp eye on all participants to see that (a) they are performing the exercises safely, and (b) they are not working too hard and showing signs of distress. Many leaders have a natural ability to gracefully and entertainingly lead the exercises. However, being a *systematic observer* does not often come naturally but is something that each leader needs to consciously develop. Systematically observing the class means that you have preestablished criteria for which you are looking in the different movements being performed. It also involves continually scanning your participants from head to toe, looking for elements of unsafe exercise technique.

The first step toward becoming an effective systematic observer is to be aware of every problem that could arise during the performance of the exercises you have selected *before* taking your place in front of the class. The easiest approach is to refer to your exercise file cards and focus on the Common Errors section. If you do not know what deviations you are looking for, you'll never see these errors. As a leader you suffer no penalty for failing to call the class's attention to unsafe movement, but you can bet the person who is exercising improperly will suffer many aches and pains as a result of your unawareness. Unless this person is redirected, he or she will continue to suffer in silence, believing in the *myth* ''no pain-no gain,'' or will eventually quit with a negative attitude toward aerobic exercise.

It is important that you observe participants in all of the following areas where problems could occur:

- Showing signs of physical distress
- Performing dance steps
- Performing exercises
- Performing locomotor skills
- Exercising with faulty posture

Continually scanning participants from head-to-toe as class is progressing is the only way you can detect and correct movement errors. Get into the practice of observing participants at different times throughout the class.

Break It to Them Gently

Another consideration of systematic observation is how to give feedback to participants about what you are observing. It's important to provide positive feedback when the class is performing the exercises safely. More important, however, is *what* you say and *how* you say it when you observe a participant performing an exercise incorrectly. When you see someone who is performing an exercise unsafely, do not confront this individual personally, for this will only embarrass him or her; plus, it shows poor leadership behavior on your part. Instead, take this opportunity to remind the entire class about exercising safely. Be specific in your comment so that the exercise can be corrected, yet be casual, perhaps even humorous, and direct your comment to the entire class. This will serve as an immediate reminder for the person(s) incorrectly doing the exercise to change and will also reinforce the proper method for everyone else.

Continuous, positive feedback tells the entire class that you are very interested in their personal safety and well being. This constant attention lets them know you care, and it also helps prevent future complaints about aches and pains.

Selecting Aerobic Dance Steps
A, B, C (Easy as 1, 2, 3)

Steps from jazz, social, folk, square, tap, and modern dance can liven up any aerobic dance-exercise class. The number of dance steps you choose to include in each routine and in each class is up to you. To achieve a fun balance of dance steps to exercise, you need to consider the following possibilities: Incorporating too much dance may

- slow down the pace of the class because of all the teaching time,
- make the class more like folk dance than aerobic dance,
- frustrate people who lack the coordination to catch on quickly, and/or
- make it too uncomfortable for participants who lack a sense of rhythm or a good self-concept when performing dance steps and dance movements.

In contrast, incorporating too little dance may

- reduce the variety of movements you can use in creating routines,
- reduce the educational value of the class,
- not use the beat of the music to its fullest potential, and/or
- bore participants who do not want to perform one exercise after the next.

Achieving a balanced class requires advanced preparation. An easy approach is to include one different dance step in each routine during the workout. You may also want to plan the week's classes to make sure that the same steps are not being repeated from routine to routine. Although participants do need to be given the opportunity to practice the steps, they will welcome the variety. Work hard to keep your repertoire of steps fresh and exciting. Including a variety of steps over the length of your session will keep participants challenged, surprised, and entertained.

Performing the Steps

Not all of your participants will move like professional dancers. While perfection of style is not a must, safe execution of the step is. For example, performing a step-ball change with the lead foot turned in or out may not look so bad. However, as opposed to keeping the lead foot straight ahead, this deviation will certainly take its toll in aches and pains.

Be familiar with the proper performance of each dance step you lead. Pay close attention to the Common Errors section of your file cards. Research reliable resource books for the proper performance of dance steps. The following books will help you learn about a variety of dance steps that can easily be incorporated into aerobic dance routines:

- Heaton, A. (1976). *Social dance rhythms*. Provo, Utah: Brigham Young University Press.
- Kisselle, J., & Mazzeo, K. (1983). *Aerobic dance: A way to fitness*. Englewood, CO: Morton.
- Lister, M., & Tamburini, D. (1965). *Folk dance progression*. Belmont, CA: Wadsworth.
- Sorenson, J., & Burns, B. (1979). *Aerobic dancing*. Rawson, New York: Wade.

Arm Movements

Once you have mastered the footwork, add some arm movements. Be as creative as you want when making up these movements to compliment the steps. Use the arms for balance, for fun, or to give an added upper body work-out. You can clap, snap, gently swing the arms from side to side, move them forward/backward, up/down, and do many more variations. Many leaders name the arm movements from song lyrics. For example, the arms can mimic windshield wipers during a step to the theme song from *Carwash* or can strum through a tune like "Dueling Banjos." Often, participants will remember a particular routine or step by recalling the arm movements that you made up to accompany them.

Keeping in Step With Your Participants
Step By Step

Regardless of the style of leading you choose, there are some helpful hints to remember as you are "choreographing" your moves. You do not need to be a dancer to be able to choreograph routines for your class. But like the dancer who moves with direction, every movement in your class should count, be well planned and performed, and correspond to the music you have selected.

Use a Variety of Music

The first step to good choreography is to keep in step with the needs of your participants. A variety of musical headlines were used in this book to reinforce the importance of using a variety of music in your class. Not everyone in your class will be into the "Top-40" hit parade tunes that so many leaders repeatedly use. Add variety by including Broadway show tunes; many of them were written especially to be danced to, so they usually are toe-tapping numbers. Also, consider both country and bluegrass music, which move participants to clap and shout as they exercise. Standing still to Earl Scrugg's "Foggy Mountain Breakdown" is almost impossible. Classical music lends itself nicely to warm-up and cool-down exercises and even to the workout. Listening to music without lyrics can be quite relaxing and hence can aid in cooling down. Movie sound tracks are full of inspirational songs, especially those from movies with athletic themes such as *Rocky*, *Chariots of Fire*, and so on. Folk songs from the 1960s will bring a smile to many participants' faces; songs by Peter, Paul, and Mary are familiar to many of us. Jazz, soul, and the Motown sound can add fun and pleasant memories to any aerobic dance-exercise class. Experiment and you'll be surprised how your own musical taste may broaden.

Use a Variety of Movements

Different types of music will evoke different senses of movement. When planning, vary the locomotor movements (walk, jog, run, hop, leap, slide, gallop, march) you use, the direction of the movement (forward, backward, to the left side, to the right side, up, down, diagonally), the arm movements (push, pull, figure eights, pointing, clapping, snapping, circling, punching), and dance steps (cha-cha, polka, grapevine, two-step, charleston, pony, swim, schottische, square dance, disco). A general guideline to follow in your planning is, the faster the music, the smaller the steps; the slower the music, the larger the steps (and the more space used).

Record All of Your Music on One Tape

Tapes are much easier to use than record players for several reasons: They are easy to stop and start in the same place; they are portable and easy to store; and they allow you to record exactly what you want to use, which makes for efficient and smooth transitions from song to song. It is also more convenient for you and less annoying to your participants if you record the music for your class on one tape. This prevents the delay of stopping and changing tapes. It also makes your preparation easier because you do not have to wind an assortment of tapes to the exact songs you intend to use. Keeping a back-up tape handy in case the other one breaks is a good idea.

Match the Musical Energy to the Exercise Energy

Be conscious of the rhythm and timing of the music. Some basic aspects of rhythm to consider are (a) the *tempo*—the pace (slowness or fastness), (b) the *meter*—how the song is organized into measures, and (c) the *beat*—the notes per measure receiving certain emphasis or accents. When listening to music, everyone has a tendency to clap on the accented beats, or when dancing, to move on these beats. If you rush your exercises ahead of the timing of the music, or lag behind it, you will end up moving to a pattern that doesn't quite fit. This off-beat movement will cause physical and mental confusion for participants. It is important, therefore, to pattern your exercises on the strongly felt beats (Scarantino, 1984).

Once you select a song you wish to use, listen to it several times. Tune in on rhythms, on repetitive parts of the song, and on any odd sections (i.e., two drum beats before the chorus). Most songs are arranged with an introduction, verse, and chorus. Also take note of any musical cues that might help you, for example, if an electric guitar is strummed four times prior to the chorus. The majority of popular music used in aerobic dance-exercise classes is written in 4/4 time, which means that each measure contains 4 beats.

When counting out the number of beats, count in sets of 4 or 8 (i.e., the introduction of a song is comprised of 6 sets of 8 beats each). Match the exercises-dance steps to the number of counted beats. For instance, let's say a song's introduction consists of 4 measures of 4 beats. You need to plan 4 sets of 4 different exercises or dance steps—that is, 4 counts of jogging forward, 4 counts of jogging backward, 4 steps of the grapevine step to the right, and 4 counts of the grapevine step to the left. A good rule to follow is to fill in any odd beats with jumps and/or claps. Always remember to figure out the footwork first and then add the arm movements. Establish a rule the first session that each new dance step always starts on the right foot; this will eliminate having to give any cue. Keep all of the exercises and steps as simple as possible. Teaching complex movement series can slow down the pace of the class and can frustrate participants who don't catch on quickly. On the other hand, if you have had the same group of exercisers for several sessions, more complex movement patterns can add enjoyment and variety.

Check your pulse upon completing the routine to monitor the intensity. Write down the routine as you work out each part for future reference. Figure out a simple notation scheme to help make writing down your routine fast and clear. For example, you could write out the words to the song on the top line, the beats on the next, and the exercise on the bottom line

I	Don't	Want	To	Walk	With	Out	You
1	2	3	4	1	2	3	4

Walk forward 4 counts   Backward 4 counts

Practice performing the routine several times and then practice leading it. If you have the chance, practice teaching it to one other person before teaching it to the class.

Dance and Exercise

You need to guard against conveying to participants that the dance steps are a "learn it and let yourself go" part of class. Although dancing adds diversity to the exercises, it is still exercise. The same mechanics that apply to safe exercising apply to doing the dance steps. For example, a participant's posture during a dance step is equally as important as his or her posture doing a bent-knee sit-up. Be familiar with the elements that comprise safe exercising and that save many participants from potential aches and pains.

Safe Exercises
Bend Me, Shape Me

A number of commonly performed exercises should be eliminated from your repertoire. These exercises serve no purpose in terms of increasing your participants' fitness levels; plus, they can cause strains and injuries. Before we examine these *risky* exercises let's learn a few terms that frequently appear in the literature to describe joint motion. Without an understanding of these terms, applying what you have read on proper exercise performance to your class will be difficult. Some common terms used to describe joint movement include the following:

Flex—Bending; decreasing the amount of joint angle

Extend—Straightening; increasing the amount of joint angle

Hyperflex—Bending beyond the natural range of motion

Hyperextend—Straightening beyond the natural range of motion

Rotation—Moving in a circular pattern

Prone position—Lying or leaning face down

Supine position—Lying on the back; face upward

Range of motion—Movement about a joint

Stabilizers—Muscles that act to hold a joint in position

These terms describe movement concisely. Learn these terms, and use them frequently in class to better prepare participants to comprehend exercise performance literature.

Exercises to Avoid or to Modify
The Safety Dance

Warm-up, workout, and cool-down exercises should focus on developing the following major muscle groups and joints of the body. Let's examine each of the following areas according to some do's and don'ts (risky exercise) when selecting safe exercises:

- Neck
- Back
- Chest, shoulders, and arms
- Hips and stomach
- Upper and lower leg
- Ankles and feet

The Neck

Take care when selecting exercises for the neck because of the potential risk of damaging the cervical vertebrae and the generally weak muscles that comprise this area. Many leaders are still having participants perform neck rolls (or circles) as shown in Figure 4.1(a) as part of their warm-up and cool-down exer-

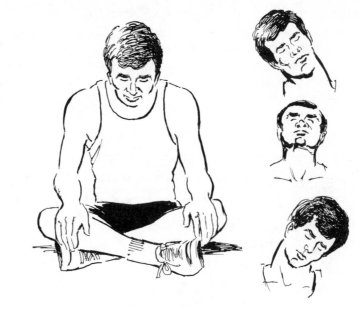

Figure 4.1(a) Neck rolls or circles—an exercise to avoid

cises. Neck rolls or circles are risky because the arching motion as the head is rolled back places unnecessary pressure on the cervical discs. This backward motion also increases the stretch of the muscles in front of the neck while contracting the back muscles of the neck. In general, the front muscles of the neck do not need stretching and the back neck muscles are already too tight.

Neck rolls or circles can be replaced with neck stretches as shown in Figure 4.1(b) and (c). To properly stretch the neck muscles, straighten up your neck in

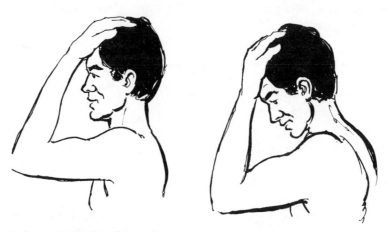

Figure 4.1(b) Safe neck stretches forward

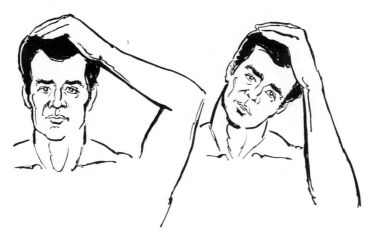

Figure 4.1(c)   Safe neck stretches to the side

a long vertical line to lessen the normal curve in the back of your neck. Relax your face and jaw, and carefully move your chin toward your neck. Lower your head toward your chest, keeping your jaw relaxed and your mouth slightly opened. Place one hand on the top back of your head; gently and continuously pull your head forward and down. Do not let your chin actually touch your chest. Feel the stretch pull all along the muscles of the back of your neck. Move your head a little to each side as if saying no, holding each tipped position for 30 seconds to a minute (Alter, 1983, p. 30).

As shown in Figure 4.1(c) return your head to a vertical position and curve your head sideways to the left, ear over the shoulder. Let your face stay looking forward, not up or down. Place your left hand on the right top side of your head and gently pull your head toward your left shoulder. Relax both shoulders and keep them down. Hold this position for 30 seconds to a minute (Alter, 1984, p.31).

In summary for the neck:

- Do *not* do neck rolls or circles.
- Do neck stretches.
- Do *not* hyperextend the neck while you are lying face on the floor or are in an ''all fours'' position.
- Do tuck your chin before performing exercises that use circling motion in the upper body or forward bending.

The Back

The back is a potentially troublesome area for many participants. You can help participants by correcting one of the most common causes of back pain—

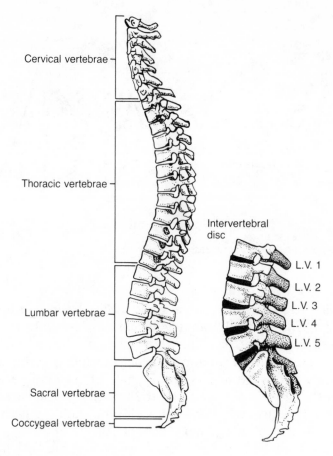

Cervical vertebrae

Thoracic vertebrae

Intervertebral disc

Lumbar vertebrae

L.V. 1
L.V. 2
L.V. 3
L.V. 4
L.V. 5

Sacral vertebrae

Coccygeal vertebrae

Figure 4.2 The spine

improper exercises. As seen in Figure 4.2 the spine consists of 33 vertebrae, stacked one on top of the other. The intervertebral discs that separate each vertebrae serve as shock absorbers and give the spine its flexibility. Two situations that play havoc with the spine are placing undue pressure (from the body's weight) on it and standing with faulty posture (see p. 71). Shown in Figure 4.3 are some popular exercises that have the potential to do more harm than good for your participant's back.

In summary for the back:

- Do *not* arch the back by any type of back bend.
- Do forward, curved, slow stretches for the back.

The Chest, Arms, and Upper Body

When performing stretching exercises or adding arm movements to a workout routine, the safety rule to remember is to take it easy. Many arm motions

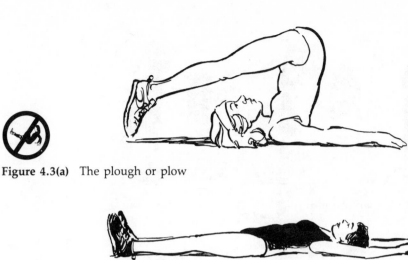

Figure 4.3(a) The plough or plow

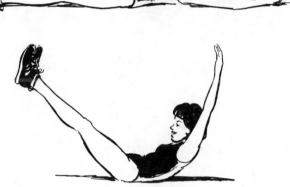

Figure 4.3(b) The V-sit

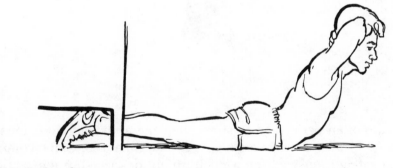

Figure 4.3(c) Back arches

used (e.g., large arm circles) take the shoulder joint beyond its natural range of motion as shown in Figure 4.4. Swinging the arms is a result of momentum and can stress the ligaments in the joints. Very little or no muscle action is actually taking place. The outermost point of the swing can even have the same effect on the muscle as bouncing (Alter, 1983).

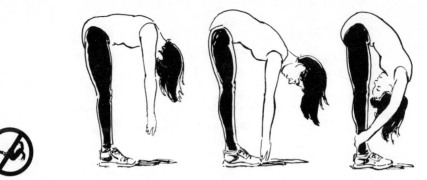

Figure 4.3(d) A straight-legged toe touch

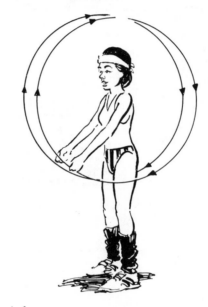

Figure 4.4 Too large of arm circles

Push-ups are often performed to strengthen the arms and chest muscles. Push-ups should also be done in a slow, controlled manner. Some common problems with safety in performing a push-up are described in the captions for Figures 4.5 a and b.

In summary for the chest, arms, and upper body:

- Do *not* do fast, uncontrolled large arm swings.
- Do controlled, smaller arm circles.
- Do *not* perform push-ups at a fast pace.
- Do push-ups in a slower, controlled manner.

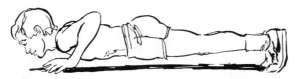

Figure 4.5(a) In a safe push-up the buttocks remains slightly raised in relation to the rest of the body to protect the lower back. The arms are never fully extended or locked on the way up. The fingers are spread to better support the body's weight.

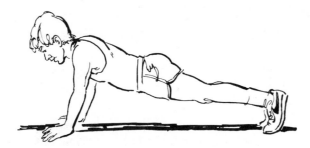

Figure 4.5(b) In an unsafe push-up the buttocks is in alignment with the body. The arms are locked as the body is raised up. The fingers are side by side making it harder for the wrist to support the body's weight.

Hips and Stomach (abdominals)

In an attempt to to lose inches from their hips and stomachs, participants will willingly engage in just about any exercise. Unfortunately, some leaders are still including prone arches, double leg lifts, and straight leg sit-ups in their reducing repertoire. The prone arch as shown in Figure 4.6 and the double leg-lift as shown in Figure 4.7 are both dangerous for the same reason. They tend to compress the discs of the lumbar spine.

The straight leg sit-up as shown in Figure 4.8(a), often performed to strengthen the abdominal muscles, also places stress on the lumbar region of

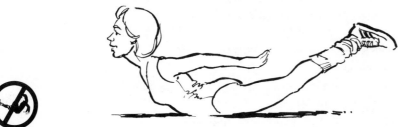

Figure 4.6 The prone arch

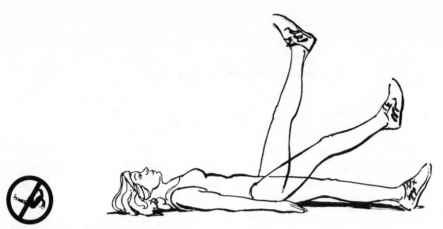

Figure 4.7   The double leg lift—either 45° or 90°

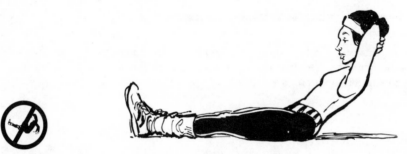

Figure 4.8(a)   Straight leg sit-ups

the spine; however, this exercise does not effectively work on the abdominal muscles. Performing straight leg sit-ups at a fast pace presents another danger: Fast action usually results in using more momentum than muscular strength and results in poorly toned stomach muscles.

The correct way to perform a sit-up is illustrated in Figure 4.8(b). A curling-up and curling-down motion is used in a bent-knee sit-up. Participants should concentrate on curling-up one vertebrae at a time, then uncurling until they almost, but do not, lie flat on the floor; then they repeat the curl-up.

In summary for the hips and stomach:

- Do *not* do prone arches or double leg lifts.
- Do *not* do straight leg sit-ups.
- Do bent-knee sit-ups in which you curl up and curl down.
- Do *not* perform sit-ups at a fast pace.
- Do perform sit-ups in a slow, controlled manner.

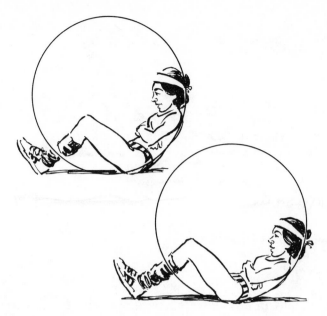

Figure 4.8(b) Curling-up sit-up

Upper and Lower Legs

The legs are continuously in motion during an aerobic dance-exercise workout. Take care to perform all of the warm-up, workout, and cool-down movements correctly. The major muscle groups of the upper leg are the quadriceps (in front) and the hamstrings (in back).

A traditional exercise to stretch out the quadriceps is the sitting Hurdler's stretch. Although this stretch can be safely performed, too often because of improper positioning, strain is placed on the knee of the bent leg. Figure 4.9(a) illustrates an incorrect Hurdler's position. Be careful not to turn the foot of the bent leg out at a 90° angle or to keep the front leg too straight. Instead, point

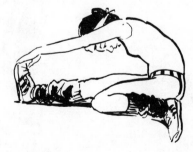

Figure 4.9(a) Incorrect Hurdler's stretch

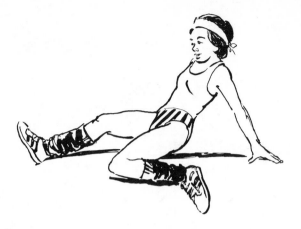

Figure 4.9(b) Correct Hurdler's stretch

the foot so that it stays in line with the bent leg, and make sure that the knee of the front leg remains bent (see Figure 4.9(b)). To stretch the quadriceps, you should lean back slowly and not lean forward, as is often the case.

A common method of stretching the hamstrings is by doing standing toe touches. Traditionally, the exercise has been performed by having participants lock their knees and try to touch their toes or the floor, as shown in Figure 4.10(a). However, keeping the knees straight or locked can place stress on the lumbar spine as you are bending forward. In Figure 4.10(b) a safer way to perform a toe touch is shown. Note that the knees are bent, the body curves down, and the elbows are relaxed.

To stretch the calf muscles safely, participants can assume the position shown in Figure 4. 11. If they slightly bend the knee of the stretching leg, they

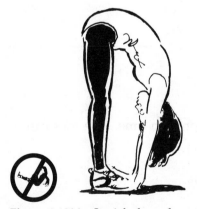

Figure 4.10(a) Straight-legged toe touch—avoid

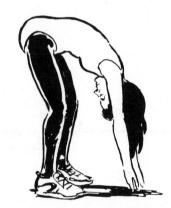

Figure 4.10(b) A safer toe touch

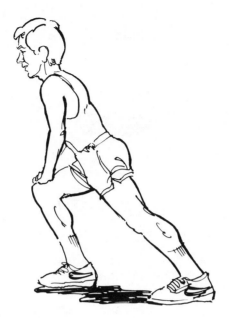

Figure 4.11 A good calf stretch

can feel the stretch. Note two important points: keeping the foot pointed straight ahead and keeping the foot squarely on the floor, as opposed to bouncing up and down.

In summary for the upper and lower legs:

- Do *not* keep the knees locked during any exercise.
- Do bend the knees as much as needed.
- Do the Hurdler's stretch correctly.
- Do *not* do any exercises that hyperflex the knees.
- Do *not* bounce while stretching.

The Ankles and Toes

Remember to do some warm-up exercises for the ankles and toes. You can warm up the ankles while sitting and doing flexions and extensions; or as shown in Figure 4.12, you can take alternating steps in place, emphasizing the transfer of weight from the ball of the foot to the floor each time. The toes can be curled up and uncurled inside the tennis shoe.

In summary for the ankle and toes:

- Do *not* forget to include exercises for the ankles and toes.
- Do include exercises for these joints in each warm-up.

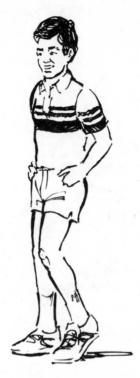

Figure 4.12 Walking in place with an emphasis on movement in the ankles

Locomotor Skills
The Locomotion

Selecting safe exercises not only applies to floor exercises or calisthenics but also to the many locomotor skills—walking, jogging, running, skipping, hopping, sliding, leaping, and galloping—so often used in aerobic dance-exercise. Never *assume* that your participants were taught the correct way to perform these skills. It only takes a few minutes of observing an aerobic dance-exercise class to see individual variations. Unfortunately, many aches and pains are still occurring because participants are incorrectly performing basic movement skills.

It is your responsibility to become familiar with the proper body mechanics of each locomotor skill. This may seem like a tall order, but this knowledge is indispensable in terms of injury prevention and safe exercise performance, for only then can you begin to detect incorrectly performed locomotor skills. For example, let's say that you are knowledgeable about proper jogging form. You are leading a routine that includes quite a bit of jogging, and you notice that a participant is continually jogging with her left foot turned out (pronated). If she continues to jog this way, the shock absorbed from the foot to floor contact will not be evenly distributed up her legs. It is only a matter of time until she complains of a painful knee or hip. As a leader, you have a choice: You could evaluate her jogging form after she complains of knee pain and wants to know why; or you could be a skillful observer, noting her deviation, and take the time to discuss proper jogging form with her, thus possibly preventing the injury from ever occurring.

In developing an understanding of each locomotor movement, you do not need a complex understanding of biomechanical principles. You do, however, need a head-to-toe idea of what the proper execution of the locomotor skill is. Because jogging is a popular locomotor skill used in many routines, let's use it as an example of how to analyze a skill (see Figure 4.13(a) & (b)).

Head—carry the head with the chin parallel to the floor. Keep the jaw muscles relaxed, not clinched. Breathe with the mouth open and at a normal rhythm, as opposed to consciously taking several deep breaths. Relax the neck muscles.

Shoulders and arms—relax the shoulders. Swing the arms at a normal rhythm in a forward and backward motion. Do not flex the elbows more than 90° degrees. Keep the hands loose but not floppy.

Hips—the hips should carry the body's weight evenly. The motion of the legs should be such that both hips can remain forward rather than rotating to the sides.

Feet—foot placement is the most important consideration in achieving good jogging form. The recommended footstrike is the heel-to-toe motion. As you

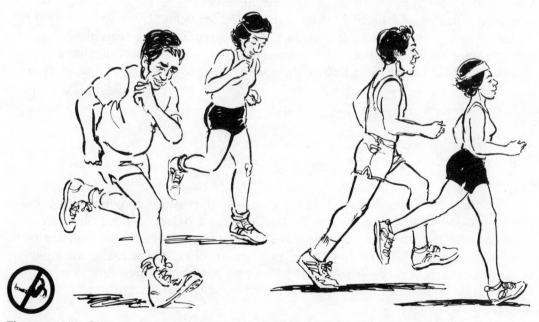

Figure 4.13(a) Improper jogging form   **Figure 4.13(b)** Proper jogging form

land lightly on the heel, the foot rocks forward to push off from the ball of the foot. If the outer border of the heel of the shoe is worn down, this indicates correct footstrike.

The following problems could result from deviations of the proper jogging form:

Head—headaches are a common problem for participants who unconsciously clinch their jaw muscles while moving.

Shoulders and arms—novice joggers will often rotate their shoulders side to side while moving. This is wasted energy and should be eliminated. Many new joggers will also flex their elbows too sharply and clench their fists as they move, which also wastes energy by increasing muscle tension.

Hips, knees, and feet—these body parts are grouped together because improper movement in one will affect the other two. For example, a jogger who throws his or her foot out to one side rather than straight ahead will force the knees and hips to absorb much more of the shock than necessary. Injuries will result if the movement is repeated often enough. Another example would be the consequences of improper footstrike. A jogger who jogs flat-footed or on his or her toes will suffer from muscle imbalances of the lower leg and could develop shin splints or other painful injuries.

Do your homework and learn the proper execution of the locomotor skills that you use most often in your routines. Several books are available to assist you in your search for analysis of movement information. I recommend that you read *Efficiency of Human Movement* (Broer & Zernicke, 1979) and *Movement Fundamentals* (Wessel, 1961). If you do not enjoy reading and searching through the literature for information, visit a biomechanist, a physical educator, a physical therapist, a trainer, or a knowledgeable aerobic specialist working in your area.

Posture
Long Tall Sally

Performing all exercises and dance steps safely requires moving with good posture. Good posture means having the body in a balanced position from front to back and from side to side. One of your responsibilites as a leader is to identify individuals who have poor posture and help them reeducate their bodies to assume a more efficient standing and sitting posture. Proper posture is the basis for effective movement, whereas poor posture contributes to fatigue.

Most muscles in the body work in pairs. For example, the abdominal muscles and the muscles comprising the lower back work together to stabilize the hip joint. If one group is weaker than the other, the hips will tilt noticeably in one direction. Becoming familiar with which muscle groups work together on one joint is important for two reasons: (a) when you plan your workout, you will be certain to balance your exercises (i.e., you would not plan 20 sit-ups for the abdomen and then neglect to do those exercises that would strengthen the lower back); and (b) when you discover a participant with posture or movement problems, you are better prepared to identify the weaker set of muscles and to help the individual begin doing corrective exercises.

General postural problems are illustrated in Figure 4.14(a). Imagine an individual with these postural problems, which is already a stress on the associated muscles, adding the stress of exercise. If a person begins with poor

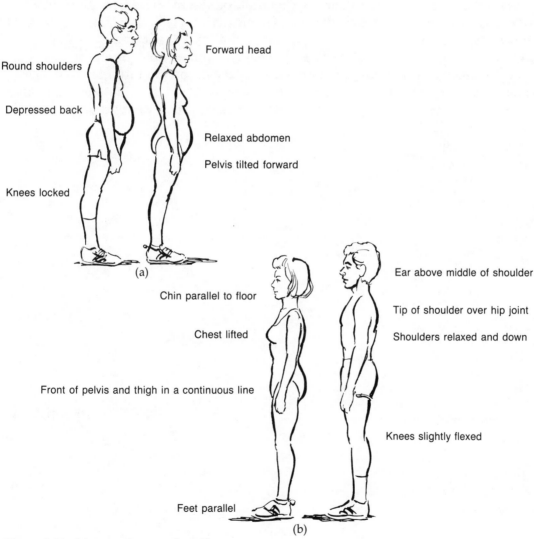

Figure 4.14 (a) general postural problems
(b) good posture

posture, exercises will only aggravate the existing problems, and the experience will be an unpleasant one. Participants who enter your class with faulty posture will unconsciously make adjustments or variations in the exercise you are leading as a result of the muscle imbalance due to their poor posture. If the body is not "carried" in a mechanically efficient form during sitting, standing, and walking, the weakened muscles of the body will be stressed as they begin to move more vigorously.

Where Do We Go From Here

After you have selected safe dance steps/exercises, have practiced leading them, and have developed your own method of systematic observation, then where do you go? It is hoped that all of your hard work in selecting, leading, and observing will pay off by eliminating or drastically reducing the number of injuries that occur during your class. However, injuries do continue to happen, and it is important that you are familiar with those common injuries that frequently plague the aerobic dancer. Different types of injuries that are common to aerobic dance and their prevention will be discussed in chapter 5.

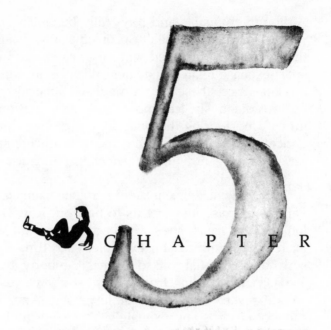

CHAPTER

Aerobic Dance-Exercise Injuries and Prevention

I Haven't Got Time for the Pain

By Melinda Flegel

Melinda Flegel is an NATA-certified athletic trainer. Melinda has a MS in physical education from the University of Illinois and taught aerobic dance-exercise in the Philadelphia area and for the University of Illinois.

Although enjoyable and physically beneficial, aerobic dance-exercise can lead to various injuries and health problems. Physicians, athletic trainers, and physical therapists are concerned with injuries in aerobic dance-exercise as well as other sport-exercise-related activities. With backgrounds in sports, medicine, and exercise science, these sports medicine specialists are well suited for affording prompt diagnosis, treatment, and rehabilitation for aerobic dance-exercise injuries. Considering the pounding, twisting, and lunging inherent in aerobic dance-exercise, you, like the sports medicine specialists, need to know how injuries happen, how to prevent them, and how to provide first-aid when they occur.

Just how stressful is aerobic dance-exercise? Biomechanists have analyzed various exercise movements to find out how they effect the body. Let's take a look at how much stress the body can be subjected to in aerobic dance-exercise. In running, for example, each time the foot hits the ground, it absorbs a force equal to 2 to 4 times the body's weight (Southmayd & Hoffmann, 1981). When landing from a leap, shock waves 4 times greater than the body's weight reverberate across the lower leg. And, in side-to-side movements, the forefoot absorbs approximately 1½ times the body's weight (Washington, Rosenberg, Friendlander, & Carlin, 1984).

We know that aerobic dance-exercise is potentially stressful, but how often do injuries actually occur? Of the relatively few studies that have been conducted, the reported injuries are fairly high. In a study performed by Richie (Richie & Washington, 1983) from 1982 through 1983, the instructors' injury rates were at 75%, while students' injuries were reported at 43%. And, in a survey of 94 instructors, Dr. James Garrick found that 55 had suffered injuries while teaching (Strovas, 1984).

With such a high incidence of injuries, the burden of class safety is put upon the leader. What can you do to minimize injuries in your class? While it is not the purpose of this chapter to teach you to diagnose and to treat injuries, it does provide you with a basic understanding of common aerobic dance-exercise injuries and health concerns—and more importantly—how to prevent them. An understanding of injuries will help you recognize potential safety problems and injuries more quickly, as well as help you to react more logically when faced with them.

Anatomical and Sports Medicine Terms

Sidewalk Talk

To fully understand the intricacies of injuries, you need to become familiar with a few anatomical and medical terms. Let's start by taking a look at the structure of a joint as shown in Figure 5.1. Knees, elbows, and other joints consist of bones, cartilage, muscles, tendons, and ligaments.

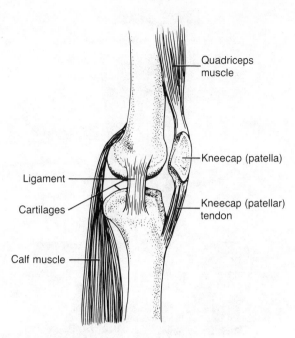

Figure 5.1 Structures of the knee joint

Muscles and ligaments are the structures responsible for holding a joint together. Ligaments act as guide wires—connecting bone to bone. With ligaments functioning as the joint's primary stabilizer, muscles serve as back-up supporters, as well as movers of the joint. Without ligaments and muscles, joints would easily dislocate or separate. Tendons connect muscles to bones and assist in making the joints move. And to protect the joints' integrity, cartilage acts as a shock absorber and prevents the bones from abrading (wearing down).

With this basic anatomy in mind, let's discuss some medical terms that you will undoubtedly come across when reading sports medicine information.

Strains—stretching and tearing injuries that affect muscles and tendons. A strain often results when a sudden or persistant stretch forces the muscle or tendon beyond its normal stretching limit. Depending upon their severity, strains can be classified in one of three categories (see Figure 5.2).

A *Grade I strain* involves stretching muscle or tendon fibers with minimal tearing. Symptoms associated with Grade I strains include little or no swelling, point tenderness at the site of injury, and mild pain when the muscle or tendon is stretched or when the muscle is contracted.

In a *Grade II strain*, a stretching of muscle or tendon fibers is accompanied by partial tearing. Grade II symptoms include pain, swelling, and possibly a slight indentation at the site of the strain.

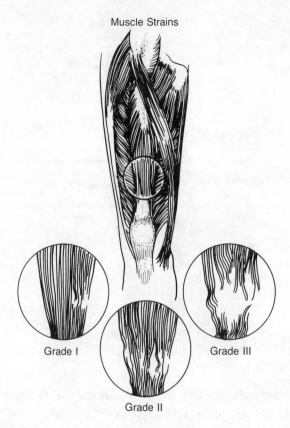

Muscle Strains

Grade I

Grade II

Grade III

Figure 5.2 Three types of strains

Grade III strains involve extensive tearing of muscle or tendon fibers and cause pain, swelling, and an obvious indentation at the injury site. Among the structures most often strained are the calf muscles, Achilles tendon, quadriceps muscles, and hamstring muscles.

Sprains—stretching and tearing injuries of the ligaments. A common cause of sprains is a sudden twisting movement that stretches or tears the ligament fibers. Sprains, like strains, can also be classified according to severity, with varying amounts of pain, swelling, and disability (see Figure 5.3).

Tendonitis—an inflammation or irritation to a tendon, resulting from overuse or from a forceful stretch. Areas most affected by tendonitis are the Achilles tendon and the elbow and shoulder tendons.

Chondromalacia—a softening or abrading of joint cartilage. It can occur as a natural part of aging (wear and tear) or as a result of a direct injury to the cartilage.

Periositis—an inflammation or irritation of the membrane that covers the bones.

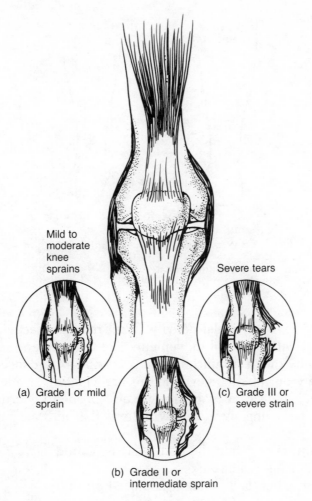

Mild to
moderate
knee
sprains

Severe tears

(a) Grade I or mild
sprain

(b) Grade II or
intermediate sprain

(c) Grade III or
severe strain

Figure 5.3 Three types of sprains

Foot pronation—a structural condition in which the foot rolls inward, under
the ankle. A normal foot is compared with a pronated or flat foot in Figure 5.4.

With the understanding of these general terms, we can now discuss some
of the specific injuries that aerobic dance-exercisers suffer.

Musculoskeletal Injuries
Hard Habit to Break

Most musculoskeletal aerobic dance-exercise injuries tend to fall into the
"overuse syndrome" category. Overuse injuries occur when the body is subjected to abnormal, constant, or repetitive stresses or when the body is inade-

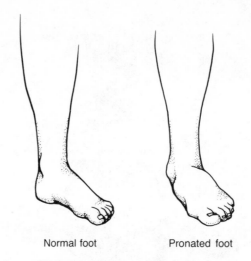

Normal foot   Pronated foot

Figure 5.4 Comparison of a normal and pronated foot

quately prepared for a particular activity. With repetitive activities like jumping and running and with stressful movements like twisting and lunging, it is easy to understand why overuse injuries can occur in aerobic dance-exercise. Individuals who are out of shape or who are participating at a level that is too advanced for their physical capabilities are also prone to overuse syndromes. Be aware of the following signs and symptoms that indicate injury:

- Persistent pain, even when the body part is resting
- Swelling and/or discoloration
- Increased pain when body weight is placed on injury
- Pain in a joint
- Pain/tenderness when lightly touched
- Deviations in normal movement patterns

The most common overuse injuries in aerobic dance-exercise include shin splints, calf muscle strain, Achilles tendonitis, bone bruises, stress fractures, and patellar (kneecap) chondromalacia. Let's take a look at each to find out why and how they happen.

Shin Splints

At the top of the aerobic dance-exercise injury list are shin splints. Both Washington et al.(1983) and Richie and Washington (1983) report shin splints as being the primary injury in aerobic dance-exercise. A catch-all phrase used to describe aching pain in the lower leg, shin splints can be caused by a strain to lower leg muscles or tendons, shin bone periositis, or stress fracture.

Causes
- Abnormal foot positioning—the foot may unconsciously tilt in (pronation) and put stress on the calf muscles and tendons.
- Muscle imbalance—the front and back lower leg muscles may not be equal in strength, causing the weaker of the two to suffer from strain.
- Excessive shock transmitted through the lower leg—unyielding floor surfaces or poorly padded shoes will force the leg to bear the brunt of impact shock.

Calf Muscles/Achilles Tendon Strain

Moving to the back of the lower leg, potential problem areas include the calf muscle and its Achilles tendon. Both injuries are felt as an aching or sharp pain, with calf strains felt in the muscle belly and with Achilles tendonitis in the upper-heel area. Standing or jumping on the toes, or rocking back or walking on the heels can be painful in both conditions.

Causes
- Shortened calf muscles or Achilles tendon—some individuals are naturally inclined to have shortened calf muscles or tendons. In others, wearing high-heeled shoes tend to let the calf muscles and tendons shorten. In either case, any stretching to the muscle or tendon beyond its normal limits can result in a strain.
- Inadequate stretching in warm-ups and cool-down.

Foot Injuries

With all the pounding in aerobic dance-exercise, it is also important to consider the foot. As in all overuse injuries, hard surfaces and improperly fitting and padded shoes can take their toll on the feet. Stress to the foot most often appears as bone bruises or arch strain.

Bone bruises and stress fractures can occur at the heel and ball of the foot. While bone bruises are commonly felt on the sole of the foot, stress fractures at the ball of the foot may often be felt on top.

Causes
- Poorly padded shoes that force the foot to absorb excess shock.
- Nonyielding floor surface that forces the foot to absorb excess shock.

Arch strain is pain felt on the sole of the foot between the heel and the ball of the foot. Most often it is a result of a strain to the tendon that spans over the area.

Causes
- Individuals with flat feet are especially prone to strains in this area.
- Inadequate arch support can also place added stress on the area.

Knee Injuries

As in the foot and ankle, the knee is also subjected to the shock of the body pounding against the floor. The most common knee problem in aerobic dance-exercise is patellar (knee cap) chondromalacia.

In patellar chondromalacia, the cartilage surface on the back of the kneecap becomes irritated and begins to crack and flake. It is most noticeable as an aching pain underneath the kneecap that is felt when climbing stairs, sitting in theaters, and in squatting, kneeling, or bending at the knee.

Causes
• Kneecap that doesn't ride properly in its groove on the thigh bone (especially in people who are knocked-kneed or bow-legged).
• Natural wear and tear on the joint from aging.
• Direct blow to the top of the kneecap.
• Excessive kneeling or squatting.

A summary of the overuse injuries and their symptoms is presented in Table 5.1.

Table 5.1 Common Aerobic Dance-Exercise Overuse Injuries

Injury	Common Causes	Symptoms
Shin splints	Abnormal foot positioning Muscle imbalance	A dull ache in the lower leg after workout
	Excessive impact shock Improper shoes	Pain on moving the foot up and down
Strains	Inadequate stretching	1st degree—some tenderness, no swelling
	Stretching muscles beyond their normal limit	2nd degree—tenderness at site, movement will be painful, swelling if not treated.
		3rd degree—immediate loss of function, swelling
Tendonitis	Inadequate stretching Repeated stress	Tenderness
Bone bruises	Hard surfaces Poorly padded shoe	Pain at the heel or ball of the foot
Stress fractures	Hard running surfaces	Pain at the fracture site
	Deviated running gait	Increase in pain with exercise
Patellar chondromalacia	Excessive kneeling/squatting Direct blow to the knee cap Knock-kneed/bowleggedness	Pain underneath the kneecap

Although strains and sprains can and do occur at the shoulders, wrists, elbows, hips, back, and neck, the incidence of these is much less than those mentioned. So let's move on to discuss a couple of general musculoskeletal problems that are more likely to occur during aerobic dance-exercise: muscle soreness and muscle cramps.

Muscle Soreness and Cramps

Muscle soreness inevitably happens to everyone in aerobic dance-exercise. Most often it occurs when individuals begin to participate either after a period of inactivity or at a higher level of difficulty. In any case, the muscles and tendons are forced to work at levels that they are unaccustomed to. The result is a general aching pain that can last anywhere from 1 to 5 days. To differentiate between muscle soreness and muscle strain, just remember that muscle strains usually have a sudden onset, are localized, and are accompanied by swelling and acute pain. Soreness, on the other hand, does not generally set in until 8 to 24 hours after exercise and is felt as a widespread, aching pain with no discernable swelling.

A muscle cramp is a painful, prolonged or spastic contraction of a muscle's fibers. It may last anywhere from a few seconds to several hours.

Causes
- Insufficient levels of potassium, sodium, or other minerals in the body. These minerals are utilized in muscle contraction, so insufficient supplies will disrupt normal muscle contractions.
- Injury or strain to the muscle or tendon.
- Insufficient supply of oxygen to working muscles.
- Fatigue.

Additional Dance-Exercise Injuries
Chances Are

In addition to musculoskeletal injuries, aerobic dance-exercisers can be confronted with other health problems. Participants can also suffer from blisters, heat illnesses, fainting, and even life-threatening conditions. A general understanding of these problems can help you make some preventive plans for your participants.

Blisters

Blisters are caused by friction between the skin and the shoe or sock and can happen to participants at any level. Friction can cause the outer and middle skin layers to rub together and, consequently to separate and fill with fluid.

Causes
- Improperly fitting shoes—too tight or too loose.
- Shoes that are constructed of an unyielding material, especially new shoes.
- Shoes with poor ventilation.

Abrasions

Abrasions, like blisters, are often caused by friction between the skin and another surface. Probably the most common abrasion in aerobic dance-exercise is the carpet burn.

Cause
- Subjecting unprotected skin to an abrasive surface, either continuously or forcefully.

Fainting

Fainting is a condition in which a participant partially or totally loses consciousness for a short period of time. Symptoms leading up to fainting may include dizziness, nausea, sweating, cold skin, and paleness.

Cause
- Lack of blood supply to the brain, resulting from fatigue, illness, injury, or shock.

Heat Exhaustion

Heat exhaustion occurs when the body is subjected to a progressive loss of body fluid through sweating. Symptoms may include profuse sweating, pale/clammy skin, headache, dizziness, nausea, fatigue, and possibly fainting.

Cause
- Failure to replace body fluids lost through sweating during vigorous activity in a hot environment. The lowered level of body fluid causes shock and circulation problems.

Heat Stroke

Heat stroke is a condition in which the body's temperature suddenly rises uncontrollably. It is characterized by hot, red, and dry skin, an extremely high body temperature, and a disruption in the sweating mechanism.

Causes
- Failure to replace body fluids lost through sweating during vigorous activity.

- Exercising in a hot, humid environment, thereby reducing the amount of perspiration that can evaporate off the body.
- Exercising while suffering from a fever.

Life-Threatening Conditions

On rare occasions a life-threatening condition such as heart failure, stroke, convulsions, or choking may occur. In the cases of heart failure, stroke, and convulsions, predisposing conditions are often the cause. Choking may occur if a student aspirates gum or candy while exercising.

Now that we know the potential injuries and health problems in aerobic dance-exercise, let's take a look at what you can do to prevent and to minimize them in your class.

Injury Prevention
You're the Inspiration

Aerobic dance-exercise or any physical activity presents a catch-22 for the body. In order to achieve fitness benefits from an activity, the body must be stressed beyond it is normal fitness levels. Still, those same stresses can injure the body if they are not properly monitored or prepared for. You can minimize injuries in your class by simply exercising a few precautions that will keep stress within healthful levels and that will protect the body against harmful stresses.

Medical History

It is a good idea to have participants complete a health questionnaire/medical history (see Chapter 7) before allowing them to participate in class. You need to be aware of any conditions that will affect their participation. Any recent injuries or health problems such as high blood pressure, diabetes, epilepsy, or heart condition warrant medical clearance for participation. You should also have seriously injured students secure medical clearance before allowing them to return to the class. These procedures will ensure your participants' safety as well as minimize your liability risks.

Surface

Floor surfaces having a combination of cushioning and stability are the most ideal for conducting classes. Cushioning is paramount in helping absorb the shock to the feet and legs, while stability is needed to provide proper amounts of traction for safe movements. Wooden, spring-loaded, and other resilient floors are preferred for their shock-absorbing capabilites. Hard, non-resilient floors like concrete and linoleum will increase injury frequency. If you must teach on floors that are unusually hard, padding or carpeting may be added to relieve the shock suffered by the feet and legs. Be sure that carpeting does not offer too much traction, however, because a surface that grabs or causes shoe drag can lead to ankle and knee sprains.

Participation

Try to keep your own instruction and student participation within healthful limits. In other words, don't overdose on aerobic dance-exercise. In Richie's (1983) study, students and instructors participating in more than three classes had a significantly higher incidence of injury. Therefore, encourage students to participate only three times a week. If you must lead more than three classes a week, use a model to demonstrate steps while you walk among the participants to systematically observe their techniques.

Experience

As mentioned in previous chapters, participants should be placed in classes appropriate to their fitness level. Ideally, the best method of instruction would be to conduct classes for specific fitness levels (beginner, intermediate, and advanced). If you lead classes containing students at a variety of fitness levels, always urge them to participate at their own pace and within their physical capabilities. A beginner could sustain a strain or overuse injury while trying to participate at an advanced level.

Technique

As mentioned in chapter 4, it is vitally important for you to practice and teach proper technique. Improperly performed or harmful exercises can lead to a whole host of injuries, including back strain, ruptured discs, and knee sprains.

Water

Make sure that participants are allowed to drink cool water periodically during class. Water intake is necessary for replacing body fluid lost in perspiration and is therefore vital to preventing heat illnesses.

Clothing

Aerobic dance-exercise clothing should be comfortable and should allow adequate ventilation. Clothing that is too tight or rough can irritate the skin, causing blisters, rashes, or even abrasions. Clothing should also be breathable, allowing evaporation of sweat. Evaporation of perspiration is necessary to help cool the body. Absolutely forbid participants to wear vinyl/rubber suits designed for weight reduction. Such suits prevent the evaporation of sweat and allow the body's internal temperature to rise. This condition can result in heat exhaustion, or worse, heat stroke.

Shoes

Shoes can play a major role in minimizing foot and leg injuries. A properly constructed and fitted shoe will aid in shock absorption and stability and will minimize blistering. Many participants will ask for some tips on how to select a good aerobic dance-exercise shoe. The following criteria (as shown in Figure 5.5) can be used when selecting and fitting shoes.

General Construction of Shoe

1. *Gradually sloping sole*—aerobic dance-exercisers land on their toes and heels and therefore need adequate padding and support in these areas. With a steeper slope from the heel to the toe, running shoes can cause toe

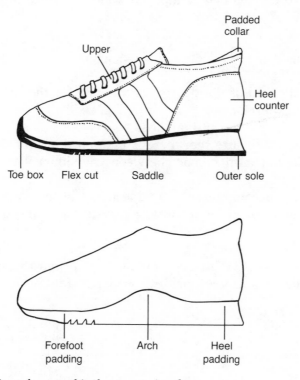

Figure 5.5 Construction of an aerobic dance-exercise shoe

problems for dancers who do a lot of hopping and lunging on the balls of the feet. Court shoes or aerobic shoes with more level soles minimize stress to the toes, yet provide enough heel lift to relieve stress to the calf and Achilles tendon.

2. *Forefoot, arch, and heel padding*—because the arch, forefoot, and heel bear the body's weight, extra padding will help absorb shock and minimize strain to these areas. Arch support is especially needed for maintaining proper foot alignment in individuals with flat or high arches or with pronated feet. If the overall shoe is good, but lacking in padding, shock-absorbing inserts can be added.

3. *Upper*—breathable material is needed to allow sweat to evaporate. Soft leather and nylon shoes allow the best ventilation. Inadequate ventilation can lead to blisters and other skin irritations.

4. *Traction*—with all the twisting and turning and starting and stopping, a good aerobic shoe should also have enough traction to prevent slipping and sliding, but not so much as to let the foot grab or drag.

5. *Flexcut*—the shoe must be flexible at the ball of the foot to allow for landing on the toes.

6. *Saddle*—the sides of the shoe should be sturdy to provide stability for side-to-side motions. A heel-counter also adds lateral stability to the heel area.

7. *Heel/ankle collar*—additional padding around the heel and ankle help to reduce stress to the Achilles tendon, as well as help to improve comfort and fit.

Proper Fit of Shoe

1. Buy shoes at the end of the day to accomodate for the gradual swelling that your foot experiences.

2. Wear athletic socks when fitting shoes.

3. At the toe box, make sure that there is enough room for the toes to fully straighten. Allow a ½-inch space between your longest toe and the end of the shoe.

4. The shoe should accommodate the widest part of the foot. Shoes that are too narrow will allow the foot to hang over the sole and can cause ankle sprains.

Using these preventative guides, you can greatly reduce the opportunities for injuries and illnesses in your classes, but what do you do if an injury does occur?

Treating Musculoskeletal Injuries
(it's got to be) Automatic

If an injury does occur in your class, you must be prepared to handle it. Beware of treating injuries, however, as you can easily leave yourself vulnerable to lawsuits. If done improperly, treatment can lead to further injury or infection. Therefore, for your participant's and your own protection as well, limit any treatment to first-aid basics.

You should obtain Red Cross certification in first aid and cardiopulmonary resuscitation (CPR). Classes are generally available from the Heart Association. Through certification you will learn how to properly care for minor injuries (scrapes, cuts, and blisters), serious injuries (fractures, bleeding), as well as life-threatening problems (heart failure, choking). First-aid classes generally require 8 to 16 hours of training, while CPR certification requires approximately 8 hours of instruction. Certification will also help protect you from lawsuits for improper treatment of an injury or illness.

Any time you suspect a serious injury or illness, you should seek medical attention immediately or suggest that the affected participant seek medical attention. Again this will help the participant as well as protect yourself from lawsuits. Is there anything you can do to initially help relieve pain and minimize further complications if any injury or illness does occur? If a musculoskeletal injury occurs during class, you can use *RICE* (rest, ice, compression, and elevation) to minimize pain and swelling.

Rest—for mild injuries, stop participation until the pain subsides. The participant can resume activity once he or she can dance without pain or discomfort. For more severe injuries, participants should rest until a physician gives medical clearance for resuming participation.

Ice—ice is an excellent treatment for minimizing pain and swelling. Always keep a cooler of ice and plastic bags available during class. Apply ice directly to the injured area for 15 to 20 minutes. Crushed ice in a plastic bag works best, because it can conform to the body. Avoid using commercial chemical ice, for it does not cool as well, and it can leave chemical burns if it is accidently punctured.

Compression—Using even pressure, wrap an elastic bandage over the ice. Start from the farthest point away from the body and wrap toward the body. For example, for the ankle, start at the toes and wrap up to the lower leg. Be sure to wrap with even pressure, yet not so tight as too cut off the circulation. Done properly, compression is effective in minimizing swelling.

Elevation—raise the injured part above the level of the heart. When used in conjunction with ice and compression, elevation helps minimize swelling.

Miscellaneous Treatment

For blisters, apply ice to reduce heat created by the friction between the skin layers. To minimize further pressure and irritation to the area, tape a donut-shaped piece of felt or foam rubber over the blister (see Figure 5.6). Do not, however, attempt to open and drain blisters. Such action, if not performed properly, may lead to infection.

For muscle soreness and muscle cramps, gradual, sustained stretching can help relax the affected muscles. Stretch the muscle for approximately 15 to 30 seconds until you can feel a slight discomfort. If performed several times, this may help relieve the pain associated with soreness or cramps.

For heat illnesses, fainting, or shock, have the participant lie down and elevate the feet higher than the head. Monitor breathing and heart rate as needed.

To learn more specifics about various treatments and how to perform them correctly, obtain first-aid and CPR certification. By applying the information and principles in this chapter you should be able to create a safe environment in which you and your participants can enjoy aerobic dance-exercise. Remember, the key to preventing injuries is to exercise caution in selecting shoes and surfaces, in organizing classes, in teaching technique, and in limiting participation. And, if an injury does occur stay calm, use *RICE*, and consult a sports medicine specialist if necessary.

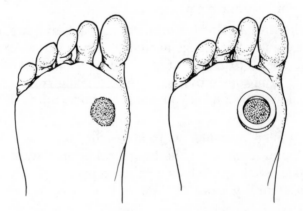

Figure 5.6 Application of a donut-shaped piece of foam rubber on a blister

You Can Depend on Me

   With proper planning you can eliminate potential aches and pains for your participants and responsibly take care of injuries if they happen. You need to evaluate your own class situation and make the best preventive and treatment plans to serve the needs of your program.

   Being well prepared to prevent and to treat injuries can make your class more appealing for participants to attend. With the high drop-out rate in classes these days, the more appealing you can make your class, the better. In chapter 6 suggestions for ways to motivate your class to attend are given.

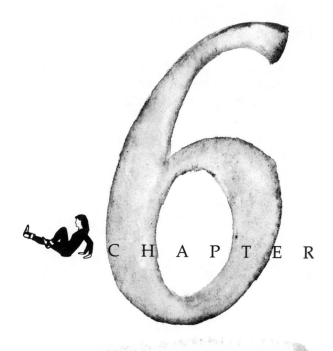

CHAPTER

Motivating Your Participants to Attend Class

Stay (Just a Little Bit Longer)

Approximately half of the people who begin an exercise program will quit within the first 6 months (Dishman, 1984). Every leader is confronted with the challenge of motivating participants to stick with his or her program. Just as your class is comprised of individuals with a wide range of fitness levels and abilities, participants also will have a wide range of psychological outlooks toward exercise. The more sensitive you are to factors that motivate participants to stick with a program, the easier it will be for you to identify participants in your class who are more likely to drop out.

Motivation is a broad term often used to describe a variety of behaviors. Motivation, in general, refers to the intensity and direction of a person's behavior. Direction of behavior means whether or not a person approaches or avoids a particular situation. The intensity of behavior relates to the degree of effort put forth to accomplish a certain behavior.

Scientists who study people's attitudes, beliefs, and personality traits in relationship to exercise are called *exercise* or *sport psychologists*. Sport psychologists examine factors that influence a person's decision to particpate in an exercise program. Most exercise scientists would probably agree that a psychological exercise prescription is not quite as easy to write as a physiological one. In this chapter you are given ideas that are the basic ingredients of psychological prescriptions geared toward motivating your participants to stick with a program. The later part of the chapter will help you think about your own motivation for wanting to be an aerobic dance-exercise leader.

Identifying Participants' Needs
Getting to Know You

> People are motivated to fulfill their needs. If you understand what your participants' needs are and if you are able to help them fulfill these needs, you possess the key to their motivation. (Martens, Christina, Harvey, & Sharkey, 1981).

How are you going to help fulfill participants' needs if you don't know what those needs are? Take the time, therefore, to get to know your participants. Try to arrive 10 minutes early and stay 10 minutes later to talk with participants about their fitness goals, jobs, interests, and so on. This also gives you an opportunity to learn what they don't like about your class. Always ask for comments in a manner that makes it easy for the participant to respond. For example, ''What is your favorite thing about my class and what one thing you would like to see changed?'' You can also take this time to encourage participants on an individual basis. Many sport psychologists will agree that one-on-one encouragement to keep exercising is much more effective than encouragement directed at the entire group.

If your class is small enough or is a captive group, such as in a corporate fitness setting, you can approach this task a little more formally by conducting a short, written survey, requesting participants' evaluations/feedback before and after each program session. Then amend your program to address those areas that need improvement.

Factors Influencing a Person's Decision to Exercise

Do It For Love

Listed in Table 6.1 are some categories that influence a person's decision to exercise. Note that the three main categories of exercise determinants are *biological*, *psychological*, and *situational* influences. These factors do not operate separately within a person. Rather a continuous, complex interaction is at work influencing decisions between these and other variables.

Biological Factors

Participants who initially have more biological advantages are much more motivated to join and to stay with an exercise program. These people are close to their ideal body weight, have a greater genetic capacity to become aerobically fit and hence see the training changes occurring faster, and have less of a predisposition to coronary heart disease. Unfortunately, the undermotivated, more overweight, less fit individual is more likely to quit. Be aware, then, that those who might benefit most from taking your class are also the most likely to drop-out.

Psychological Factors

The exercise psychologist studies the psychological traits of an exerciser through three basic approaches: attitudes, beliefs, and personality traits.

Table 6.1 Factors Influencing a Person's Decision to Exercise

Biological Traits of the Exerciser	Psychological Traits of the Exerciser	Situational Factors
Body weight	Self-motivation	Support from family and friends
Fitness level	Attitudes and beliefs	Job status
Health status	Personality traits	Location of exercise facility
		Class atmosphere

Attitudes—a person's attitude is how he or she feels or thinks about something. Participants will join your class with a variety of attitudes formed from past experiences as well as with expectations they have about your class. Although attitudes can be used to predict a person's initial involvement in exercise and the type of exercise program he or she would select, the fact that a person thinks of exercise as a positive experience is no guarantee that he or she will stay with the program (Dishman, 1984).

Beliefs—a person's beliefs about the health benefits of exercising also affects his or her participation in the program. Some strongly believe that exercise will produce many health-related benefits, while others just as strongly believe that exercise will do little for them. Most participants who enter your program with a particular health problem or with the belief that exercise will be an ounce of prevention against future health problems will probably be more motivated to stay.

Personality Traits—personality traits are those complex characteristics that distinguish one individual from another. One of the most studied personality traits in terms of exercise adherence is self-motivation. A self-motivated person is one who is reinforced more by his or her own ideas and goals than by others. Self-motivated people have a much higher success rate at staying with an exercise program. These individuals seem to be better suited to overlook things (i.e., the exercise room, the time class is being held) that other participants might easily use as excuses not to attend.

Situational Factors

Because biological and psychological traits are very personal factors, not much can be done to these motivational influences. Situational factors, however, are more easily altered in hopes of increasing your participants' motivation to regularly attend your class. How your participants react to the setting in which your class is being held, the location and convenience of accessibility to that setting, and the atmosphere in which you conduct class are examples of situational factors.

Helping a Participant to Set Goals
Day By Day

Helping individuals establish realistic exercise goals toward which to work is an important part of motivation. Many participants drop out because they expect to become instantly fit, and this does not happen. In a positive manner, warn participants of all the likely drop-out factors (e.g., hard work, pain, and time commitment). Keep encouraging participants to make the class and exercise a habit. To help reinforce making the class a habit, have participants set some realistic goals to accomplish.

Establishing short-term and long-term goals provides a participant with objectives to work toward. Goal setting is an effective means of eliciting commitment to the program. Personally discussing each participant's goals will give you the necessary insight to modify any unrealistic goals that person may have set. For example, one of your participants has set a goal of losing 20 pounds during your 8-week session. You know that exercising alone will not accomplish this goal and that 2 pounds per week ($2 \times 8 = 16$) is a safe rate of weight loss; therefore, you need to explain to this participant what he or she can expect from your class in terms of weight loss. The participant must understand that diet and exercise are the best approaches to attaining and to maintaining weight loss. The participant should set short-term goals of losing 1 to 2 pounds a week by attending your class and by reducing his or her caloric intake. At this rate, the participant may accomplish a safer, more desirable long-term goal of losing 10 to 15 pounds in 2 months. When planning goals with each participant, remember to take into account his or her physical ability, commitment, and previous success in accomplishing goals.

Offering Incentives In Your Program
Right or Wrong

Some aerobic dance-exercise programs award participants with incentives as motivation to continue attending class. Incentives, or rewards, are usually given for accomplishing certain short or long-term goals. The idea of giving *extrinsic* (external) rewards such as T-shirts, badges, and trophies must be evaluated. Sport psychologists have conducted several studies about how giving rewards may affect an individual's *intrinsic* (internal) motivation for participating in exercise. It seems that some individuals participate for intrinsic reasons such as enjoyment and fun. Others, however, are more motivated to participate for the external reward(s) attached to participating.

Rewards can be informational or controlling. Informational rewards affect a person's self-concept. For example, giving a participant the most-improved award conveys a message of achievement and improvement in his or her ability. In contrast, controlling types of awards take away a person's internal desire to participate and replace it with motivation to receive the award. For example, you could offer a free T-shirt and matching leotard to the participant who lost the most weight at the end of the session. Once a participant sets out to win the award, his or her motivation for attending your class could shift from an intrinsic one to one of the external motivation of winning the outfit.

Rewards do not always undermine a person's intrinsic motivation to participate. It all depends on how your participants interpret the awards you may decide to offer in your class. In aerobic-dance exercise, extrinsic awards should be given for participation, not for performance. This reinforces the idea of making exercise a life habit.

Providing a Pleasant Exercise Setting
I Think I'm Gonna Like It Here

Contributing to a participant's perception of an enjoyable workout environment are the physical features of the exercise room, such as furnishings, lighting, ventilation, and temperature. Although you can't always have everything you may want, due to budgetary constraints or to the design of the room, try to provide your participants with the best environment possible.

Features of the Exercise Room

Size. The amount of space in which your participants have to move around in will certainly affect your planning. Participants need enough room to stretch out their arms freely and to perform dance steps and exercises without hitting or running into others. Always seek a classroom compatible to the number of participants you anticipate having.

Mirrors. Mirrors add to the attractiveness of the exercise room and make the room appear larger. Participants will also enjoy the visual feedback as they work out. The leader can systematically observe the class without turning around. Mirrors should be of high quality so they can always continue to provide an accurate reflection (Halcomb, 1983).

Furnishings. As mentioned in chapter 4, decorate the workout room as attractively as possible. You can hang posters, fill bulletin boards with aerobic dance tips and quips, and post educational materials on training-related topics and on information participants might bring to share. Make it a point to always keep the area clean and free of safety hazards such as dirt, clothing on the floor, tracked-in water, and anything else that might be specifically related to your workout area.

Lighting and ventilation. Exercise rooms need to be well lit and well ventilated. Bright lighting will make the participants feel more alive and ready to work out. Windows are a welcome addition to any exercise facility. If space permits, use large fans or ceiling fans to aid in circulating the air.

Room temperature. Many rooms within a building or complex are controlled with a central thermostat. Pay attention to the temperature of the workout room. If the temperature exceeds a reasonable 70°, see what can be done to aid in cooling the room.

Location of the Class

The location of your class should be a convenient one for as many people signing up for class as possible; otherwise, the easier it will be for someone looking for an excuse not to exercise to find one. A person's home and work location significantly influences his or her exercise patterns. Choosing the right location to hold your class will make a big difference in the attendance. Because of this relationship between convenience and exercise adherence, many companies have developed on-site exercise facilities.

Creating the Class Atmosphere
Camelot

The atmosphere in which your class is conducted will also affect participant's motivation to attend. Try to create a comfortable, noncompetitive atmosphere where participants will enjoy working out. Encourage participants to work out at their own pace, to ad-lib, to experiment, and to have fun. As a leader you can facilitate this type of environment by always giving positive feedback and by being human yourself. Establish a positive rapport with your participants; then, when you have an off day (and you will) and make a mistake, the class will be understanding and positive toward you in return.

Being a Positive Communicator

An effective motivator is first an effective communicator. When talking with your participants, keep the following points in mind:

- Don't treat your participants as inferior or assume they are naive. Speak to them in the same way you want them to speak to you.
- Use the class's suggestions, when appropriate, to let them know that you are listening to them.
- Always be positive or provide constructive feedback. No one should be made to feel stupid by trying to do something and then being told point blank that he or she is not doing it well.
- Don't be on the defensive when participants criticize you. Try to listen and turn the conversation around into a more positive situation for everyone involved.
- Work toward being an effective communicator with other professionals involved with your program as well as with the participants.

Creating the Mood

It's a common-sense fact that the mood the leader brings into the classroom will affect the participants. An effective leader will leave his or her troubles outside of the classroom door and enter in a very uplifting mood. This is the mark of a professional. You could encourage your participants to do the same thing so that they get the most out of the session. Remind them that this is 1 hour of the day in which they can relax and do something for their mind and body.

Displaying Confidence

The level of self-confidence a leader displays to the class may influence some participants' motivation to stick with the class. Your self-confidence comes across to the class verbally and nonverbally. Verbal confidence usually takes the form of loud and clear instructions, positive comments from systematic observations, and assurance in your tone of voice as you ask and answer questions. Nonverbal confidence is usually displayed by graceful movement, by effective use of the hands to indicate changes in direction and speed, and by pleasant facial expressions as opposed to a look that conveys mild fright or indecisiveness. Being well prepared to lead can only boost your level of self-confidence.

The Effect of Teaching Styles on Motivation
Where You Lead

Many variations of aerobic dance-exercise programs have evolved since Jacki Sorenson designed her first class in 1969. Two basic styles of leading, however, seem to prevail: The routine-based style and the follow-the-leader style. Participants may feel more comfortable working out to one style than to another. How comfortable a person feels about learning by a certain style can influence his or her motivation to continue.

Routine-based programs are generally structured by having the participants learn several precisely choreographed routines. These routines are comprised of a variety of combinations of exercise and dance steps. Participants perform a series of routines each time participants come to class. These routines are usually choreographed to popular music, and many of the lyrics are used as names for the various exercises and dance steps. In some programs the leader is required to learn specific routines that an administrator of that particular organization has choreographed.

The follow-the-leader format differs in that you are not locked into teaching specific routines; nor do you repeat the same routines from class to class over the length of the session. Leaders who use this style usually choreograph their own "routines" to be used. The term *routine* is used loosely in the sense that the routine is often choreographed and performed in an impromptu manner. In some follow-the-leader programs, the music is used only for background, and the exercises-dance steps may or may not be performed to the beat of the music.

You may prefer to use a combination of these styles of teaching. Both of these approaches have something to offer and preferences depend largely on your skills, the class structure, and the participants' needs and abilities. Let's examine some of the advantages and disadvantages to each style of teaching.

Advantages of using the routine-based style:

1. You can establish a sense of continuity throughout the program using this style.
2. You can teach participants new dance steps and movement patterns and repeat sequences often.
3. You can plan a theme around each session as extra incentive for people to participate.
4. You have access to several resource records of choreographed routines that are available for novice leaders. You need to evaluate each record in terms of safe exercises, prior to using it in class.
5. You might have a greater sense of confidence teaching a predetermined routine.

Disadvantages of a routine based style:

1. You might sacrifice a continuous, vigorous work out by stopping often to teach steps.
2. You might forget to be a systematic observer by concentrating too hard on remembering steps.
3. Some participants may have problems following steps, so you must be prepared to talk to them and encourage them to keep moving and to do their best.
4. Some participants may feel that doing the same routines time after time is boring, so always try to include something new in each class.
5. If you forget the steps as you are leading, it will most likely throw off participants who closely watch you as they work out. If you use routines, instruct the class to continue moving and pick up the correct steps later in the song rather than to quit and wait for you to get back on track.

Advantages of the follow-the-leader style:

1. You don't have to teach participants a lot of steps, sequences, or patterns.

2. You are not limited to songs to which you have already choreographed routines. This means that participants can bring in their music to use.
3. You can use your creativity because no preestablished routines have been designated.
4. You can easily provide a continuous, vigorous workout.
5. You can ''improvise'' more easily as you begin to get feedback from the participants. If you have a class of highly motivated individuals, have them pool their talents, and together with your guidance, make up a routine. For instance, each participant could take a turn contributing a 4-count exercise/step and keep adding to it until the song is over.

Disadvantages of the follow-the-leader style:

1. You must work at cueing in the class for the next movement to ensure smooth transitions and a nice flow of movement.
2. You must keep the exercises-dance steps easy to follow so that participants will not have trouble following and keeping up.
3. You must still think ahead to avoid the problems inherent to ''winging it'' for the entire class. For example, you may use the same exercises and dance steps from song to song because you can't think of steps impromptu; or, you are thinking so much about what the next step will be that you do not systematically observe the class.
4. Some participants may not like not knowing what step is coming next or exactly how many times they will be performing it. Be prepared to discuss the class format with these participants.
5. Although this style allows for creativity, it also means much work, especially in situations where you have some of the same participants in your class for the entire year or when you are expected to design a new program every 8 to 12 weeks.

Do It With Style

The style of leadership you choose depends upon what you are most comfortable with and upon what you are capable of doing. It also depends on which style you enjoy teaching most. If you've only used one style, experiment and try a combination of the two. Lead a few routines so that each time a particular song is played, the class knows what to do. You can then spend more time systematically observing. Also include a few follow-the-leader free style classes. For variety, ask participants to suggest a few exercises you can evaluate and use. Further, involve participants by asking them which style they prefer. Finally, whenever you get the chance, observe other leaders' teaching styles. All of these methods will help you develop a style that works best for you.

Examining Your Own Motivation
Should I Do It?

Besides considering what you can do as a leader to motivate your participants, it is important to think occasionally about what motivates you to want to be a leader. These factors might include such things as prestige, acquiring teaching experience, personal enjoyment, and/or the salary. Pinpointing your own reasons for wanting to be an aerobic dance-exercise leader may not be that easy, however, as Friendenberg (1959) stated,

> Self-appraisal is not a simple task . . . What we must decide is perhaps how we are valuable rather than how valuable we are; the question is more qualitative than quantitative. We learn fairly accurately how we look through (other's) eyes but if we are at all wise we learn not to see ourselves through their eyes, but rather to accept their image of us as our guide to be considered in establishing our conception of ourselves . . . Self-esteem is therefore closely related to clarification of experience: if we do not understand clearly what we have done and what has happened to us, we have no true basis for self-esteem. (pp. 106-107)

Take the time to identify your reasons for wanting to teach aerobic dance-exercise. As you identify key motivating factors, ask yourself how these factors could affect the quality of the job you will perform as a leader. Do these factors have a positive or negative effect on the job you do as leader? Arriving at answers to this question will help you become a better leader.

> A leader is best
>   when people are least aware of his leadership;
> Not so good
>   when people acclaim and obey him blindly;
> Worse
>   when they despise him.
> But of a good leader
>   who talks little,
>   when his work is done
>   and his aim fulfilled,
> They will say,
>   ''We did this thing ourselves''
>
> Lao-ste   (ca.565 B.C.)

The Leader as a Role Model
Let's Get Physical

Whether you like it or not, as an aerobic dance-exercise leader you are a role-model for many of your participants. The stereotyped fitness instructor is perceived as being physically fit, is at his or her proper body weight, and is able to perform the dance steps and exercises quite well. Often, this stereotype may also include that the aerobic dance-exercise leader doesn't smoke, drink alcoholic beverages in excess, eat junk food, or indulge in any other "unhealthy" behaviors.

How you perceive yourself as a role-model depends upon your own philosophy. There are many professional variations when it comes to identifying what comprises a good role-model. Take time to formulate your own beliefs and attitudes; then you will be ready to discuss them intelligently if the subject ever comes up in class or when you are talking with other leaders. Your participant's perception of you as a role model can or cannot be a motivating factor. That is, if a participant expects you to be in top shape and at your body weight, and you are neither, that participant may question the benefit of taking your class.

Leader of the Pack

Motivating participants to stick with your program is a real challenge. Getting to know your participants and their needs will help you tailor your program to meet these needs. Each program setting will bring with it different kinds of individual concerns. By becoming involved with your participants, your ability to motivate them to stick with your program will improve markedly.

Planning some motivational strategies will pay off with better attendance. Likewise, planning and taking care of some administrative duties will enhance the benefits received from everyone involved in your program. In chapter 7 you will learn about a few administrative duties you need to take care of prior to leading your first class.

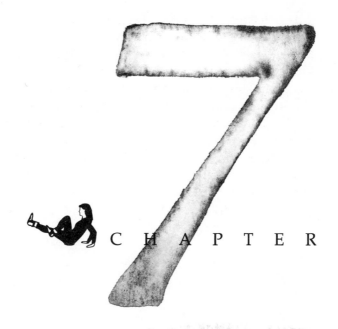

7

C H A P T E R

Administrative Notes for Aerobic Dance-Exercise Leaders

It's Up to You

The preceding chapters have given you some guidelines and principles from the exercise sciences. Applying these guidelines will make your program safer, and more well rounded and enjoyable for participants. In addition to knowledge from the exercise sciences, you need to consider a few administrative duties in your planning. If you are a leader in an established program, chances are good that these administrative procedures are taken care of already. Your role, then, becomes one of understanding what is expected, of carrying out these procedures in the classroom, and of giving the administration some input from your practical classroom experiences. If you are a self-employed leader, you must attend to these responsibilities yourself. Just as your class benefited from the guidelines applied from the exercise sciences, your overall program will benefit from attending to these administrative tasks. The following tasks are discussed in this chapter:

- Legal liability
- Advertising
- Program ideas
- Salary considerations
- Program evaluation

Legal Liability
Risky Bizness

By law, you are required to fulfill certain responsibilities for your participants' welfare. You owe your participants certain "duties." Whether or not you comply to these duties will be of utmost importance should a participant get injured in your class and file a lawsuit. The following legal duties were adapted from the American Coaching Effectiveness Program's text titled *Coaches Guide to Sport Law* by Gary Nygaard and Thomas Boone (1985). The duties have been modified to apply to an aerobic dance-exercise class.

Using Proper Technique

As you know by now there are proper and improper ways of structuring your aerobic dance-exercise class. For example, there are rules governing format (warming up, working out, and cooling down), proper exercise-dance step selection, the appropriate frequency, intensity, duration, and so on. Failure to lead the class in a safe, progressive exercise program is infringing on your participants' rights to trust you as a knowledgeable leader.

Hand in hand with teaching proper exercise-dance techniques is warning participants about what could happen if they do not follow your instructions. For example, let's say that you just explained the physiological rationale for progressing in the intensity, frequency, and duration of a workout. However, you do not warn participants that if they exceed their predetermined intensity, distressful symptoms may stop their workout altogether. All explanations of the proper ways to exercise should be accompanied with appropriate warnings of what could happen if participants don't follow your instructions.

Adequate Supervision

The importance of systematic observation was stressed earlier in this book. You owe it to your participants to continually be on the lookout for improper dance-exercise techniques and signals of overexertion. You should never leave participants unsupervised for any reason. Supervision means that you are in charge, so it is your responsibility to be there and to be ready.

Sound Planning

Obviously, the goal of an aerobic dance-exercise class is to have participants achieve certain training benefits. Progression toward this goal must be done slowly and with preestablished increments to meet the fitness level of the group you are leading. Sound planning means that you have covered how you will handle everything, from providing a safe exercise room and leading safe routines, to having thought about how you would handle an emergency. Sound planning encompasses planning for each of these duties and more.

Inherent Risks

Participants need to be told the inherent risks involved in taking an aerobic dance-exercise class. Inherent risks are risks that accompany all types of exercise/fitness classes. For example, aerobic dance-exercise is a vigorous form of exercise that carries the risk of potential muscular and cardiac problems. Generally speaking, an inherent risk is one incurred in a normal class, working out in a safe facility with a qualified instructor. The qualified instructor is aware of, understands, and does everything in his or her power to minimize the dangers of inherent risks.

Just as you warn participants about improper exercise technique, you must also warn them against inherent risks. Take the time to discuss inherent risks with participants the very first meeting and to repeat the warnings periodically.

Safe Workout Environment

The more sensitive you are to creating a safe workout environment, the better off your participants will be. Before class begins, check the room for any unsafe conditions. In an aerobic-dance exercise class this includes such items as water on the floor, a newly waxed floor, dirt, uneven surfaces, and poor ventilation. Inspect the workout environment every day prior to class.

Teaching in a gym could present additional problems: for example, support beams in the middle of, or at the end of the floor, projections hanging down from the ceiling, or equipment left sitting out from other classes. Warn participants to stay off all equipment, and point out the potentially dangerous construction features of the room. Before working out in any setting, do not forget to consider the temperature of the room as a safety factor.

Proper Training

Lack of knowledge does not protect you when your are faced with a liability suit. The better prepared you are and the more carefully you carry out the proper training techniques, the safer you will be in case of an emergency situation.

Health Records and Fitness Test Results

Ideally, before participants join your class, they should have filled out a medical history form and should also be handing you the results of a series of fitness tests they have undergone. Based on this information, your job of placing these individuals in the appropriate level of exercise class and providing them with some educational information on their personal health needs would be much easier. Most exercise programs do not yet have the luxury of having individuals undergo extensive fitness tests before joining a class; however, it is still your responsibility to obtain as much information as possible from each person in terms of health status and fitness data—prior to participating in your class.

Health records—each program needs to have a tailored health status report to keep on file for each participant. This report should contain information on the person's current medical problems, risks of medical problems, signs and symptoms of health problems, and an assessment of his or her lifestyle health behaviors (e.g., exercise patterns and nutritional habits). Several standard health risk appraisal forms, which you can modify, are available to provide you with important participant information. This information will alert you to the special needs of an individual; also it will contain any necessary referrals for that person prior to joining your class: For example, if someone reports that they have severe asthma, then you need to get a doctor's clearance before that person can participate in your program. You can also use this information to prepare your minilectures on educational topics. Keep all of the information confidential.

Fitness data—if every participant prior to joining your class gave you his or her test results from a graded exercise stress test and a muscular fitness test, you would have plenty of information to prescribe an individualized workout.

Then you would know where this person needs to improve and what kinds of goals could realistically be set. More and more fitness leaders are learning how to administer these tests, and someday this will indeed be the case for all leaders. In the meantime, however, many individuals have access to gaining this information outside of your class, for example, at a YMCA or a university or an adult fitness center. Give participants the opportunity to inform you of all the fitness data they may have acquired before joining your class, and keep this information confidential as well.

The more information you obtain from your participants and the more you use this data to tailor their workouts, the safer program you will obviously have. If you are interested in becoming qualified to obtain health status information and to administer fitness tests, contact the American College of Sports Medicine for requirements of becoming a Health/Fitness Instructor.

First Aid and Emergency Plans

How well your first aid and emergency system works depends upon you. Prepare in advance how to effectively handle injuries or accidents. You need to be able to provide first aid and to establish a plan to secure emergency medical help when necessary. In a situation demanding first aid, it is important to know that you will be held negligent if you do nothing. You will be just as negligent if you select the correct procedure and perform it incorrectly.

You should be trained to administer first aid and cardiopulmonary resuscitation (CPR). Check your skills periodically to review them and to renew your certification. Keep a well-supplied first-aid kit on hand. If possible, have access to another room where first aid can be given. Also, make plans as to what will take place once a participant becomes injured. For example: Will class be over? Will someone lead for you?

In circumstances where a person is in need of further medical treatment, have a plan of action prepared for contacting medical personnel. Your plan will depend upon your available resources. For example, you might call the university health center, a private physician, the emergency squad, or and in-house physician with whom you have made prearrangements. Have this person(s)' telephone number accessible at all times, and be prepared to give a complete description over the phone. The more details you can provide, the better.

Record Keeping

Keep a written record of the cause of the injury and of the specific care you provided. Accident report forms can be obtained from the National Safety Council. When you fill in the report, keep it simple yet thorough. Record the information completely, precisely, accurately, and objectively. A written report will help you recall the facts of the case should a participant decide to press charges against you. Evaluate the accident or injury to determine the cause or contributing factors. Once these factors are identified, work toward correcting or eliminating them from your program.

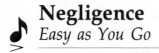

Negligence
Easy as You Go

If a participant sues you, and your case is brought to trial, the judge and jury will be examining your behavior in light of fulfilling the duties mentioned. The most common lawsuit brought against fitness leaders is one of negligence. Negligence means that you failed to act as a reasonable and prudent leader. In attempting to determine that you were negligent, the judge and jury have to prove the following four factors:

1. *Presence of the Duty.* Did you owe the participant the duty in question? (More times than not you did.)
2. *Breach of Duty.* Was that duty unfulfilled (breached)? (Did you do the proper thing but do it incorrectly?)
3. *Cause of the Injury.* Was it your breach of duty?
4. *Extent of the Injury.* What was the actual extent of the injury?

All four factors must be proven before you can be found negligent. If any one of the factors is missing, liability cannot be charged.

Waivers

Many programs have participants sign waiver forms to release the leader from liability in the event of an injury. However, do not rely too heavily on waivers as protection from liability because most courts will not allow a person to waive his or her rights in the event of negligence.

Liability Insurance

Check to see if the program in which you are working provides you with any type of liability insurance. If not, it is advisable to have a clause added to your personal insurance policy that will protect you if necessary. Several professional organizations offer reasonable liability insurance for instructors. For example IDEA (International Dance Exercise Association) offers a liability package to its members.

Summary

Participating in aerobic dance-exercise classes has its risks, and it is your responsibility to reduce those risks. Meet the challenge of your responsibilities by thinking through your entire program, giving maximum attention to the welfare of your participants. Know your legal duties prior to leading your first class. The more qualified you are, the better your position should someone decide to sue you.

Advertising Your Program

Who Will Buy?

The way you advertise your program may make quite a difference in the number of people who attend your class. If you are a leader in an established program, the advertising and promotions for that program have been taken care of already. Nevertheless, always be on the lookout for new ideas to add to current marketing strategies. But if you are self-employed, advertising your class becomes a major concern.

The two main things to consider in advertising your program are (a) the cost involved and (b) the amount of your time invested. It is hoped that the money and the time spent on advertising will be proportional to the number of people you attract to your program. *Demonstrations, written ads,* and *word of mouth* are possible advertising strategies. Their success depends upon the amount of time and money you can afford to devote to them.

Demonstrations

Demonstrations can be a successful means of advertising. You can plan a 10 to 20 minute demonstration designed to educate your audience about aerobic dance-exercise. During this time your audience can also experience participating. Your demonstration can consist of one warm-up routine, one moderately paced workout routine, and one cool-down routine. Prior to leading participants in each routine, you can explain the format of your class and the rationale for its structure. At the close of the demonstration, allow time for questions.

During your demonstration time, you must impress the audience of the following: that you know what you are talking about, that you are easy to follow, and that they can gain benefits from participating in your program. You have to sell them on the idea that participation is fun, beneficial, and worth the time and money they are investing.

Good planning is the key factor in a successful demonstration. Be sure to communicate to whomever is in charge of the arrangements exactly what you will expect the participants to do. There is nothing more unsettling than to plan on having a group to workout with you, then to show up at the facility in a T-shirt and shorts and to find out that your audience is attired in work clothes. You also need to inquire about what equipment and space is available for use. Showing up with a box of tapes to play at a place that only has a record player will quickly put a damper on your presentation. Arrange to have chairs stacked against the wall, and equipment moved so that you will have all the available space possible for your workout.

Use your imagination for planning effective demonstrations. For example, perform with a small group at the half-time of a popular sporting event or designate a special night in a school gymnasium. Some businesses might even be receptive to the idea of a lunch-time demonstration for employees.

Written Ads

Written ads can take the form of flyers, newspaper advertisements, folded notices, and so on. When writing the ad, include all of the pertinent information concerning your class: for example, your credentials, the fitness level of the class, location and what benefits participants can expect to gain. Make flyers attractive and, if possible, professionally made at a print shop. Post them in strategic locations geared toward the audience you are trying to reach and leave them posted until class gets underway.

If you are trying to reach employees of a certain company, get permission to have your folded notices stuffed in with their paychecks. Most businesses have a centrally located lounge facility that contains bulletin boards for notices, flyers, and other items of interest for employees. Posting flyers will help reinforce the notices the employees received with their paychecks.

Newspaper ads will cost so much per line depending upon your community. These ads can be effectively coordinated with your other means of advertising.

Guest Days

Designating a certain day or days each month as guest day can increase people's awareness of your program. But exercise caution if you choose to let guests participate in the workout. Remember that these people may have never attended an aerobic dance-exercise class prior to yours. To let them workout without knowing how to take their heart rate and without being familiar with other class procedures would be quite foolish. Establish a special guest day routine. New exercisers can then get a feel for the entire working format of class and for the overall goals you and the class are working toward accomplishing.

Word of Mouth

Perhaps the best kind of free advertising is by word of mouth. Have persons in charge of groups you are interested in reaching make announcements about your program. You'll need to prepare these brief, concise announcements and see that they are delivered to the appropriate person.

People who have taken your class before are good sources of free advertising. Personal testimonials of the fitness and fun derived from your class will be just as effective (if not more) than all of the written ad copy you can generate. Do not overlook the possibility of having people in your class go out and recruit with you.

Salary Considerations
She Works Hard for Her Money

Before deciding to work for a certain salary, you should consider several variables. For example, a contract offering you $12 dollars an hour might sound appealing; but as you begin subtracting program-related expenses (i.e., the gas used driving back and forth to the exercise site, tapes, liability insurance), the offer may begin to lose some of its appeal. In whatever type of work setting you select, find out what is included in your salary, as well as how the management fixed that rate. Then when preparing to discuss your salary, consider competitive rates and your experience and qualifications.

The Aerobics & Fitness Association of America conducted a 6-month survey in their journal *Aerobics & Fitness* to collect information on instructor wages. Figures 7.1 and 7.2 display their findings as reported in May/June of 1985.

Competitive Rates

Some established programs at colleges, universities, and recreation departments pay their leaders minimum wage, or slightly above. While this may sound disappointing, do not discount the experience and job references gained from working in these programs. Being a leader in a well-organized program offers rewards that outweigh financial gains. You will learn good organizational tips, good managerial skills, and worthwhile knowledge about safe exercise programs from the experienced people in charge of these programs. Because of the large number of people who apply to be leaders, these programs often expect a great deal from their leaders, yet pay them minimum wage. Some programs, however, pay minimum wage because of budgetary constraints.

If you decide to work for a privately owned aerobic dance-exercise program, inquire about salary and the costs you will be expected to cover yourself in the interview stages of applying for this job. For example: Are you expected to drive long distances to get to your class? How many hours a week are you being asked to teach? Do you have to provide any equipment (tapes, player) for your program? This is the time to discuss all of your concerns and all of the company's policies affecting your salary.

If you are going to be a self-employed aerobic dance-exercise leader, you will be responsible for calculating your own budgetary expenses. A good start-

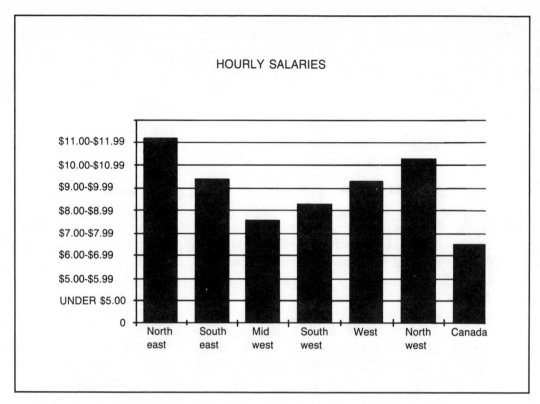

Figure 7.1 Aerobic dance-exercise instructors' hourly salaries. Note: From *Aerobics & Fitness*, May/June 1985, Vol. **3**, No. 3, (p. 38) by Aerobics and Fitness Association of America. Reprinted with permission.

ing point is to check around town and find out what your competitors are charging for their classes. Be sure that your rates include any overhead costs (i.e., room rental, lighting, equipment) that apply to your class.

Your Experience and Qualifications

Your experience and qualifications for teaching aerobic dance-exercise should be taken into account during salary negotiations. A more experienced and qualified leader is generally a more confident and safer leader to employ. Your experience and qualifications will lend credence to the program and hence, probably inspire greater attendance. You deserve to share in the profits that are being generated because of your abilities as a leader. Bring your years of experience and your qualifications to your employer's attention. Possessing certain training or certification when applying for the job or acquiring such while you are teaching, may or may not be justification in your employer's opinion for a raise (Aerobics & Fitness, 1982).

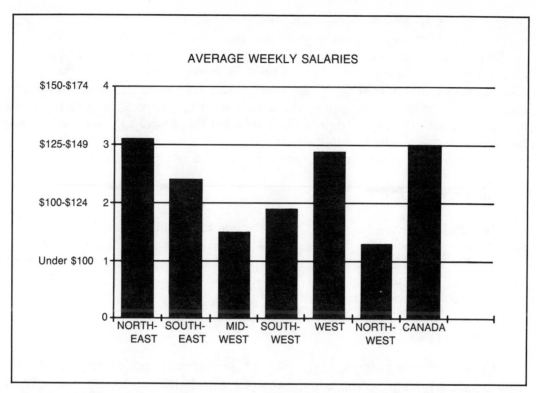

AVERAGE WEEKLY SALARIES

Figure 7.2 Aerobic dance-exercise instructors' average weekly salaries. Note: From *Aerobics & Fitness*, May/June 1985, Vol. **3**, No. 3, (p. 38) by Aerobics and Fitness Association of America. Reprinted with permission.

Program Ideas
These Are a Few of My Favorite Things

Observing other leaders' classes and sharing ideas with them can give you some ideas to try in your own program. Here are some practical ideas from other leaders that you might find useful in your program.

Planning a Program Theme

Many private and corporate aerobic dance-exercise programs are set up to run for 8-, 10-, or 12-week sessions. The leader might choose a theme for each session around which the routines are designed. To add to the fun you can have T-shirts made for the participants, select songs that go with the theme, and decorate the dance room to match the theme. Examples of themes could include "The All American Woman," "The Fifties," "Let's Get Physical,"

"Great American Movie Heroes and Heroines," and so on. If you are teaching in a corporate setting, you can personalize the theme to go with the company.

Themes work well for smaller classes, attended by the same participants each week. They do not work as well in larger recreational settings where classes are usually offered on a "walk-in" basis. Themes often can increase the incentive to participate because of the anticipation to see how creative the leader can be about sticking to the theme. You want to be sure to plan out the entire program before offering to lead; otherwise, it could require searching midway through the session for some songs you don't already have.

Magic Carpet Ride

One leader provided her class with squares of carpet, donated by a local carpet store, to use during floor exercises. When it was time for floor exercises, participants helped themselves to the carpet squares, kept stacked up in front of the room, and put them back when they finished. (Several participants volunteered for carpet squares laundry duty.)

Monitor

If you have a large class, you may wish to hire someone to help you in your job of systematic observation. Someone who is trained to look for signs of distress and to correct erroneous execution of exercises is a valuable asset to the safety of your program. This person(s) can also encourage participants and help them monitor their heart rate. Both you and your participants will appreciate a monitor who is well trained and has a good personality.

The Dance Connection

With the popularity of aerobic dance-exercise today, it's not unusual to find many programs being offered within one community. In a few cases the leaders of different programs have arranged to meet 2 days a year so that they can exchange ideas and resources. However, leaders are often uneasy about initiating such a meeting out of fear that their program will appear inadequate in comparison to others. Take the initiative to arrange a meeting and invite everyone on the premises that no program is better than another and that every leader has something to offer and something to learn; and you will find that these meetings will be extremely exciting and productive for everyone who attends.

Educate as You Decorate

It was mentioned earlier that as part of a theme it's fun to decorate the workout room. Participants will always enjoy coming to a bright, clean, well-lit room to work out. Take this opportunity to educate your participants. Make attractive posters containing information on exercise-related topics such as nutrition, effect of weather conditions on exercising, fluid replacement, and heart rate. Add a dash of humor by including topics such as Erma Bombeck's columns on attending aerobic dance-exercise or cartoon strips about aerobic dance-exercise classes.

Preparing an Exercise Reference List

Posters, charts, and pictures help create a pleasant workout environment and serve to reinforce important concepts the class needs to know. They might even stimulate participants to ask questions about exercising that they hadn't thought of before. It isn't necessary for you to be an expert on all of the related topics of exercise and fitness. However, you should be able to refer participants to *reliable* sources of information they can read on their own. These sources should be written in nontechnical, understandable language. If you are not sure you can compile such a reference list, use the ones provided here or seek out experts in your community who are likely to assist. Such community help might come from experts located at universities, schools, hospitals, YMCAs, private physicians, volunteer agencies, and so on.

The following is a list of possible topics of interest about which your participants might ask. You and your participants can add to this list. Some popular topics might include the following:

1. The energy systems
2. Components of physical fitness
3. Fitness appraisal
4. Heart disease—hypertension
5. Medical exams before beginning an exercise program
6. Weight-lifting programs
7. Smoking and exercise
8. Flexibility and stretching exercises
9. Environmental concerns and exercise
10. Body composition and weight control
11. Nutrition and exercise
12. The menstrual cycle and exercise
13. Shin splints and common injuries
14. Stress and exercise
15. Lower back problems and exercise
16. Training programs and guidelines
17. Safe exercises
18. Diabetes and exercise
19. Pregnancy and exercise
20. Ergogenic aids

Once participants express an interest in reading about a topic, you need to point them toward some reliable reference books. The following list of books was selected because their accurate information is written in easy-to-understand terms. Here's how to use the list. Each book on the list covers some or many of the topics on the popular topics list. If the topic is discussed in the reference book, the number of the topic appears underneath the title of that book. For example, Gabe Mirkin's book contains information on the energy systems (1), components of physical fitness (2), heart disease (4), weight lifting (6), flexibility exercises (8), environmental concerns (9), body composition (10), nutrition (11), training programs (16), safe exercises (17), and ergogenic aids (20). This book, therefore, would be referenced as follows with the corresponding numbers in the list:

Mirkin, Gabe. (1976). *The Sportsmedicine book*, Boston: Little Brown.
   *1, 2, 4, 6, 8, 9, 10, 11, 13, 16, 17, 20

All the reference books have been matched to the topics they cover. Although this list is not an all-encompassing one in terms of available fitness books, each represents a good source for participants to learn more information and is a good starting place for their search for more knowledge.

Cailliet, Renee. (1981). *Low back pain syndrome* (3rd ed.). Philadelphia: F.A. Davis Company.
   *15
Dilfer, Carol. (1977). *Your baby, your body*. New York: Crown Publishers.
   *17, 19
Fox, Edward, and Mathews, Donald. (1981). *The physiological basis of physical education and athletics* (3rd ed.). Philadelphia: Saunders College Publishing.
   *1, 2, 3, 4, 5, 6, 7, 8, 9, 10, 11, 12, 13, 14, 16, 17, 19
Getchell, Bud. (1979). *Physical fitness: A way of life*. New York: John Wiley & Sons, Inc.
   *1, 2, 3, 4, 5, 6, 7, 8, 9, 10, 11, 12, 14, 15, 16, 17, 18, 19, 20
Jacobson, Edmund. (1978). *You must relax*, (5th ed.). New York: McGraw Hill.
   *14
Katch, Frank. (1983). *Nutrition, weight control, and exercise* (2nd ed.). Philadelphia: Lea & Febiger.
   *1, 2, 3, 4, 5, 6, 7, 8, 9, 10, 11, 12, 14, 15, 16, 17, 18, 19, 20
Melleby, Alexander. (1982). *The Y's way to a healthy back*. Piscataway, NJ: New Century.
   *8, 14, 15, 16, 17

Selye, Hans. (1976). *The stress of life* (revised edition). New York: McGraw Hill.
*14

Sharkey, Brian. (1984). *The physiology of fitness* (2nd ed.). Champaign, IL: Human Kinetics.
*1, 2, 3, 4, 5, 6, 7, 8, 9, 10, 14, 15, 16, 17

Sims, Dorothea. (1984). *Diabetes: Reach for health and freedom* (revised edition). St.Louis, MO: The C.V. Mosby Company.
*1, 4, 5, 7, 9, 10, 11, 14, 16, 18, 19

Wells, Christine. (1985). *Women in sport: A physiological perspective*. Champaign, IL: Human Kinetics.
*2, 3, 5, 9, 10, 11, 12, 16, 19, 20

Williams, Melvin. (Ed.) (1983). *Ergogenic aids in sports*. Champaign, IL: Human Kinetics.
*11, 20

Evaluating Your Program
Reflections

To measure the degree of success of your program, you must conduct periodic (every 6 to 8 weeks) evaluations. Use all available data to determine how you are doing in each area of your total program. You need to be able to honestly evaluate such questions as, Are the participants attending your class on a regular basis? and, Are they enjoying themselves? If the answer to these questions is no, then what will be your plan of action for making improvements?

To evaluate your program, you need to make a checklist of each important aspect. The following sample checklist can be used as a starting point to establish one that meets your own needs. You will need to adapt certain areas of this sample to meet the needs of your program. For example, in Part II: Exercise Environment, classes are conducted in a variety of settings. You will need to consider the special features of your own facility when planning your evaluation.

When evaluating your program, fill out a checklist yourself and also ask one other person whose opinion you value to complete one. Then get together and compare notes on how your program is going and identify the strong areas of your program and those that need improvement. You may even want to get a selected amount of participant feedback by evaluations as well. Then more input you can get, the better your program will continue to be.

Program Evaluation Checklist

Part I: Leader Qualities

Indicate your strengths and weaknesses in each of the following areas. For each checkmark in the ineffective column, outline a plan of action for improvement.

Category	Effective	Ineffective
Effective communicator with:		
Younger participants	_____	_____
Same age participants	_____	_____
Older participants	_____	_____
Other staff members	_____	_____
Resource contacts	_____	_____
Effective motivator with:		
Younger participants	_____	_____
Same age participants	_____	_____
Older participants	_____	_____
Physically fit participants	_____	_____
Beginning level participants	_____	_____
Confidence level in front of:		
Younger participants	_____	_____
Same age participants	_____	_____
Older participants	_____	_____
Other staff	_____	_____
Teaching style:		
Routine-based	_____	_____
Follow-the-leader	_____	_____
Combination	_____	_____
Rapport with:		
Younger participants	_____	_____
Same age participants	_____	_____
Older participants	_____	_____
Resource contacts	_____	_____

Other:

Comments for improvement:

Part II: Exercise Environment

Indicate the appropriate rating in each of the following areas of your exercise environment.

Safety:	Safe _____	Unsafe _____
Cleanliness:	Clean _____	Unclean _____
Lighting:	Well lit _____	Poorly lit _____
Ventilation:	Well ventilated _____	Poorly ventilated _____
Room temperature:	Too cool _____	Too warm _____
Location:	Convenient _____	Inconvenient _____
Atmosphere:	Cheerful _____	Dreary _____

Other:

Comments for improvement:

Part III: Class Format

Rate the segments of your class format and make the appropriate changes.

Warm-up exercises:	Offer variety _____	Little variety _____
Workout routines/moves:	Offer variety _____	Little variety _____
Cool-down:	Offer variety _____	Little variety _____
Relaxation exercises:	Include _____	Do not include _____
Beginning and ending class on time:	On time _____	Late _____
Musical selection:	Offer variety _____	Little variety _____
Educational material:	Include _____	Do not include _____

Other:

Comments for improvement:

Part IV: Legal Liability

Place a checkmark in the appropriate area and make plans for improvement.

Insurance:	Adequate _____	Inadequate _____
Techniques:	Proper _____	Improper _____
Supervision:	Adequate _____	Inadequate _____
Planning:	Sound _____	Unsound _____
Inherent risks to participants:	Identified _____	Unidentified _____
Workout environment:	Safe _____	Unsafe _____
CPR and first aid:	Certified _____	Uncertified _____
Health records and fitness data:	Available _____	Unavailable _____
Emergency plans:	Established _____	Unestablished _____

Other:

Comments for improvement:

Part V: Budget and Salary

Place checkmarks in the appropriate areas and make any necessary plans for improvement.

Advertising:	Cost effective _____	Not cost effective _____
Salary:	Adequate _____	Inadequate _____

 Reachin' for the Sky

Whether you are self-employed or a part of an aerobic dance-exercise staff, give each class everything you've got. Work hard to achieve a safe, enjoyable program for your participants. Stay up-to-date, keep smiling, and continually reach for the sky. If you are always prepared to lead, to observe, to learn, and to be yourself, you'll be a successful aerobic dance-exercise leader.

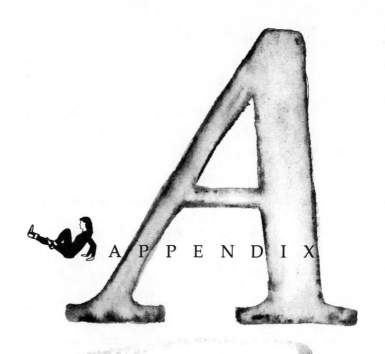

A P P E N D I X

**Resources to
Keep You
Up-to-Date**

Magazines

Aerobics & Fitness

This magazine contains a broad spectrum of articles on health and fitness. The Aerobics and Fitness Association of America is actively involved in certification of aerobic dance-exercise leaders. The magazine is published bimonthly by:

Aerobics & Fitness Association of America
15250 Ventura Blvd.
Sherman Oaks, CA 91403

Corporate Fitness

An informative journal for any leader working within a corporate fitness program. It contains articles on all aspects of aerobics and fitness programs. This journal is published bimonthly by:

Barrington Publications, Inc.
825 S. Barrington Avenue
Los Angeles, CA 90049

Dance-Exercise Today

A trade magazine for the dance-exercise professional. Each issue features several articles on aerobics, jazz, and all forms of exercise set to music. This magazine is published 6 times a year by The International Dance-Exercise Association (IDEA). IDEA is currently involved in the issue of instructor certification.

IDEA
4501 Mission Bay Drive Suite 2-F
San Diego, CA 92109

The Physician and Sportsmedicine

This journal is written for practicing physicians and professionals interested in the medical aspects of exercise, sports medicine, and fitness. It is published monthly by:

McGraw-Hill, Inc.
4503 W. 77th Street
Minneapolis, MN 55435

Women's Sport and Fitness

This magazine contains the latest news on nutrition, dance-exercise, running, and other fitness topics of interest. It is published 11 times a year by:

Women's Sports Publications
P.O. Box 612
Holmes, PA 19043

Newsletters

Healthline

A newsletter published monthly as a nonprofit public service by the Fredrick Burke Foundation and San Francisco State University. It contains articles on preventive care topics and fitness related information.

Healthline
1320 Bayport Ave.
San Francisco, CA 94070

Nutrition and the M.D.

Different nutritional topics are explored in each issue of the newsletter. It is sponsored by UCLA as a continuing education service for physicians and nutritionists. It is published by:

PM, Inc.
P.O. Box 2160
Van Nuys, CA 91404-2160

Running and Fitness (a newspaper)

The recreational athlete's newspaper of health and fitness ideas. It contains information compiled from interviews, research, and personal experiences on the benefits of diet, exercise, play and other fitness topics. It is published bimonthly by:

American Running & Fitness Association
2420 K Street NW
Washington, DC 20037

Sports Medicine Digest

This newsletter contains material on the prevention, treatment, and re-habilitation of sports injuries. It also contains information on nutrition, fitness, and upcoming sports medicine related symposiums. It is published monthly by:

PM, Inc.
P.O. Box 2160
Van Nuys, CA 91404-2160

The Harvard Medical School Health Letter

This newsletter provides accurate and current health information written for the general public. It is published monthly by the Department of Continuing Education of Harvard Medical School.

The Harvard Medical School Health Letter
P.O. Box 2438
Boulder, CO 80302

The Tufts University Diet and Nutrition Letter

This contains recent information on health and nutrition. It is published monthly by:

Tufts University Diet and Nutrition Letter
P.O. Box 34 T
322 West 57th Street
New York, NY 10019

Catalogs

Consumer Information Catalog

This paper-back booklet lists booklets from almost 30 agencies of the Federal Government. More than one-half of the booklets are free and the rest are available for low or reasonable prices. Booklets are available on a host of topics ranging from health care and exercise to how to fix your car and buy a house. It is published four times a year by:

Consumer Information Center
Dept. H
Pueblo, CO 81009

Hoctor Products

This catalog contains products for dance and physical education. It features a wide selection of records, books, manuals, teaching aids and equipment for physical educators. A catalog is available from:

Hoctor Products
159 Franklin Turnpike
Waldwick, NJ 07463

Kimbo Educational

This catalog contains records and cassettes for all types of dance and exercise for all ages and fitness levels. Catalogs are available from:

Kimbo Educational
P.O. Box 477
Long Branch, NJ 07740

Team Aerobic Dance Handbook

The Amateur Athletic Union has published the rules to participate in competitive team aerobic dance. For further information write to:

AAU House
3400 W. 86th Street
P. O. Box 68207
Indianapolis, IN 46268

Aerobic Dance-Exercise Organizations

Aerobics and Fitness Association of America
15250 Ventura Blvd., Suite 802
Sherman Oaks, CA 91403

American Alliance for Aerobic Exercise Instructors, Inc.
368 8th Street
Brooklyn, New York 11215

American College of Sports Medicine
P.O. Box 1440
Indianapolis, IN 46206

Fitness Resources
RFD #3 Box 198
Concord, NH 03301

International Dance-Exercise Association
4501 Mission Bay Drive, Suite 2-F
San Diego, CA 92109

National Dance-Exercise Instructor's Training Association
1503 Washington Ave. South, Suite 208
Minneapolis, MN 55454

The Aerobic Center
12200 Preston Road
Dallas, TX 75230

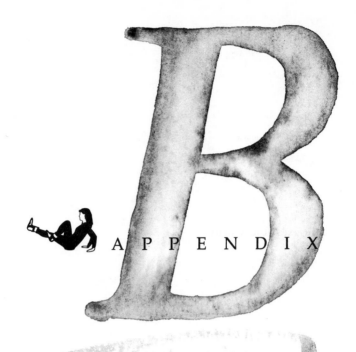

APPENDIX

Song Titles

Song Title	Artist	Album	Suggested Use
Chapter 1			
I Hope I Get It	Company	A Chorus Line—Original Soundtrack	Workout
It Might Be You	Dave Grusin	Soundtrack to Tootsie	Warm-up
I Dowanna' Know	Reo Speedwagon	Wheels Are Turning	Workout
Nature of the Game	Christopher Cross	Another Page	Warm-up
Ease on Down the Road	Michael Jackson	Soundtrack to the Wiz	Workout
Chapter 2			
The Body Shop	Barbara Streisand	Soundtrack to the Main Event	Workout
If	Bread	The Sound of Bread	Cool-down
We Go Together	Soundtrack to Grease	Soundtrack to Grease	Warm-up
With Every Beat of My Heart	Laura Branigan	Self-Control	Warm-up
You're the One	The Oak Ridge Boys	Y'all Come Back Saloon	Warm-up
And Every Breath You Take	Sting	Dancing Greatest Hits	Warm-up
I Could Have Danced All Night	Audrey Hepburn	Soundtrack to My Fair Lady	Workout
I Want Muscles	Diana Ross	Silk	Warm-up
Light My Fire	José Felicianó	Encore	Cool-down
I Sing the Body Electric	Soundtrack to Fame	Soundtrack to Fame	Warm-up
How Sweet It Is	James Taylor	Greatest Hits	Warm-up
Chapter 3			
That's the Way I've Always Heard It Should Be	Carly Simon	Greatest Hits	Cool-down
Prepare Ye	Soundtrack to Godspell	Soundtrack to Godspell	Warm-up
Let Them Work It Out	Sergio Mendés		
Take It Easy	Eagles	Eagles Live	Workout
Stormy Weather	Frank Sinatra	LA is My Lady	Cool-down
We've Only Just Begun	Arther Fiedler/Boston Pops	Greatest Hits of the 70s	Warm-up
Chapter 4			
Best That You Can Do	Christopher Cross	Soundtrack From Arthur	Warm-up
Both Sides Now	Judy Collins	The Best of Judy Collins	Warm-up
Follow Me	John Denver	Greatest Hits	Cool-down
Private Eyes	Daryl Hall & John Oates	Private Eyes	Workout
A, B, C	Jackson 5	A, B, C	Workout
Step By Step	Al Jarreau	Jarreau	Workout
Bend Me, Shape Me	The American Breed	Unknown	Workout
The Safety Dance	Men Without Hats	Dancing Greatest Hits	Workout

(cont.)

128 LEADING AEROBIC DANCE-EXERCISE

Song Title	Artist	Album	Suggested Use
The Locomotion	Grand Funk Railroad	Greatest Hits	Workout
Long Tall Sally	The Beatles	The Beatles Live	Workout
Where Do We Go From Here	Barry Manilow	Even Now	Cool-down
Chapter 5			
I Haven't Got Time for the Pain	Carly Simon	Hotcakes	Warm-up
Sidewalk Talk	Jellybean	Mix Up	Workout
Hard Habit to Break	Chicago	Chicago 17	Cool-down
Chances Are	Johnny Mathis	Greatest Hits	Cool-down
You're the Inspiration	Chicago	Chicago 17	Cool-down
Automatic	Pointer Sisters	Break Out	Workout
You Can Depend On Me	The Manhattan Transfer	Manhattan Transfer	Workout
Chapter 6			
Stay	Jackson Browne	Running on Empty	Workout
Getting to Know You	Soundtrack to The King and I	Soundtrack to The King and I	Warm-up
Do It for Love	Sheena Easton	Do You	Workout
Day By Day	Soundtrack to Godspell	Soundtrack to Godspell	Warm-up
Right or Wrong	Wanda Jackson	Country Hits of the 60s	Warm-up
I Think I'm Gonna Like It Here	Andrea McArdle	Soundtrack to Annie	Workout
Camelot	Richard Harris	Soundtrack to Camelot	Warm-up
Where You Lead	Carole King	Tapestry	Warm-up
Should I Do It?	Pointer Sisters	Black & White	Workout
Let's Get Physical	Olivia Newton-John	Physical	Workout
Leader of the Pack	Bette Midler	Divine Madness	Workout
Chapter 7			
It's Up to You	John Denver	Back Home Again	Cool-down
Risky Bizness	Kris Kristofferson	Easter Island	Cool-down
Easy As You Go	Carmen McCrae,	Take Five Dave Brubeck	Cool-down
Who Will Buy?	Soundtrack to Oliver	Soundtrack to Oliver	Warm-up
She Works Hard for Her Money	Donna Summer	She Works Hard for Her Money	Workout
These Are a Few of My Favorite Things	Julie Andrews	Soundtrack to The Sound of Music	Warm-up
Reflections	Soundtrack From Rocky	Soundtrack From Rocky	Cool-down
Reachin' for the Sky	Peabo Bryson and Roberta Flack	Live & More	Cool-down

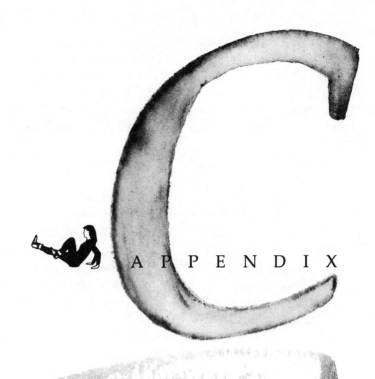

APPENDIX

Aerobic Dance-Exercise Articles and a Suggested Reading List

Leaders in aerobic dance-exercise programs, as well as scholars studying aerobic dance-exercise from a research-oriented point of view, are always looking for the latest articles. To aid in this search, this appendix lists articles that have appeared in all types of journals from the very scholarly to the more lay publications. To assist researchers looking for articles from aerobic dance-exercise studies these articles will be marked with an asterisk (*).

Anshel, M. (1985, April). Aerobic dance for athletes. *Athletic Journal*, 16-18.

Barton, B.J. (1982, March). Aerobic dance and the mentally retarded: A winning combination. *Physical Educator*, **39**, 25-29.

Chiles, B.A., & Moore, S. (1981, February). Aerobic dance in public schools. *Journal of Physical Education and Recreation*, 52-53.

*Clearly, M.L., Moffatt, R.J., & Knutzen, K.M. (1984). The effects of two- and three-day-per week aerobic dance programs on maximal oxygen intake. *Research Quarterly for Exercise and Sport*, **55**, 172-174.

Cohen, A. (1984, March). Dance-aerobic and anaerobic. *Journal of Physical Education, Recreation and Dance*, 51-53.

Dielens, S. (1984). Narcissism and fashionable physical activities: Psychological profile of aerobic dancers, joggers, and bodybuilders. *Revue de L'Education Physique*, **24**, 21-25.

*Dowdy, D.B., Cureton, K.J., DuVal, H.P., & Ouzts, H.G. (1985). Effects of aerobic dance on physical work capacity, cardiovascular function and body composition of middle-aged women. *Research Quarterly*, **56**, 227-233.

*Durrant, E. (1975). *The effects of jogging, rope jumping, and aerobic dance on body composition and maximum oxygen uptake of college females.* Doctoral dissertation, Brigham Young University, Salt Lake City, Utah.

Farnell, L. (1984). The use of aerobic dance as a conditioning tool for sport. *Sports Coach*, **7**, 8-11.

Fitness Report. (1984). Am I dancing as fast as I can? *American Health*, **3**, 28.

Fitnews. (1985 March/April). Toxic aerobics. *Fitness Management*, 14.

Foster, C. (1975, March). Physiological requirements of aerobic dancing. *Research Quarterly*, **46**, 120-122.

*Francis, L., Francis, R., & Welshons-Smith, K. (1985). Aerobic dance injuries: A survey of instructors. *The Physician and Sportsmedicine*, **13**, 105-111.

Furman, A. (1983, November/December). Aerobic dance injuries. *Running and Fitness*, 18-19.

Gearson, R.F. (1985, December/January). Checking out aerobic dance. *Corporate Fitness and Recreation*, **4**, 26-29.

Halcomb, R. (1983 October/November). Introducing a class act. *Corporate Fitness and Recreation*, 37-43.

Halcomb, R. (1985 December-January). Making room for aerobics. *Corporate Fitness and Recreation*, **4**, 24-25.

Hibsch, M. (1984). National certification standards: A clear solution. *Dance-Exercise Today*, **2**, 20-21.

*Hooper, P., & Noland, B. (1984). Aerobic dance program improves cardiovascular fitness in men. *The Physician and Sportsmedicine, 12,* 132-135.

*Igbanugo, V., & Gutin, B. (1978). The energy cost of aerobic dancing. *The Research Quarterly, 49,* 308-315.

Kerr, K. (1984, February). Aerobic dance: A consumer's guide. *Journal of Physical Education, Recreation and Dance,* 55, 50-51.

Kuntzleman, C., & Runyon, D. (1985 March/April). Profitable teaching. *Fitness Management,* 34-35.

*Legwold, G. (1982, September). Does aerobic dance offer more fun than fitness? *The Physician and Sportsmedicine, 10,* 147-151.

McCabe, M.G. (1982, September). Ask before you dance. *The Physician and Sportsmedicine, 10,* 150.

*Metcalf, J.A., Watson, H.K., Matthews, R.G., & Guynn, C.H. (1981). ECG effects of aerobic dance. *Postgraduate Medicine, 70,* 219-223.

Nash, H. (1985, October). Instructor certification: Making fitness programs safer? *The Physician and Sportsmedicine, 13,* 142-155.

Perry, P. (1984). Dancing on the job. *American Health, 3,* 28.

*Read, M.T.F. (1984). Runner's stress fractures produced by an aerobic dance routine, *The British Journal of Sports Medicine, 18,* 40-41.

Richie, D.H., Kelso, S.F., & Bellucci, P.A. (1985). Aerobic dance injuries: A retrospective study of instructors and participants. *The Physician and Sportsmedicine, 13,* 130-135.

Rockefeller, K.A., & Burke, E.J. (1979). Psycho-physiological analysis of an aerobic dance programme for women. *The British Journal of Sports Medicine, 13,* 77-80.

Russell, P.J. (1983, October). Aerobic dance programs: Maintaining quality and effectiveness. *Physical Educator, 40,* 114-120.

*Slenker, S. (1982). Effectiveness of aerobic dance and bicycle ergometer programs for female employees. *American Association of Business and Industry, 5,* 4-5.

Strovas, J. (1984). Aerobic dance teachers are not injury proof. *The Physician and Sportsmedicine.* 12, 24.

Taylor, E.B. (1985, March/April). Aerobic certification: What's it worth? *Fitness Management,* 53-54.

Tipton-Empey, G. (1985, May). Aerobic exercise. *National Raquetball,* 22-25.

Vetter, W.L., Helfet, D.L., Spear, K., & Matthews, L.S. (1985). Aerobic dance injuries. *The Physician and Sportsmedicine, 13,* 114-117.

Weber, H. (1974). The energy cost of aerobic dancing. *Fitness for Living, 8,* 26-30.

References

Aerobics & Fitness. (1985, May/June). Sherman Oaks, CA: The Aerobics and Fitness Association of America.

Alter, J. (1983). *Surviving exercise.* Boston: Houghton Mifflin.

Broer, M., & Zernicke, R. (1979). *Efficiency of human movement.* Philadelphia: W.B. Saunders.

Dishman, R. (1984). Motivation and exercise adherence. In J. Silva, III, & R. Weinberg (Eds.), *Psychological foundations of sport* (pp. 420-435). Champaign, IL: Human Kinetics.

Foster, C. (1975). Physiological requirements of aerobic dancing. *The Research Quarterly, 46,* 120-124.

Fox, E.L. (1983). *Lifetime fitness.* Philadelphia: W.B. Saunders.

Friedenberg, E. (1959). *The vanishing adolescent.* New York: Dell Publishing Company, Inc.

Garrick, J.G., Gillien, D.M., & Whiteside, P. (April, 1985). *The epidemiology of aerobic dance injuries.* Paper presented at American College of Sports Medicine. Vol. 17, No. 3.

Gerson, R.F. (1985). Checking out aerobic dance. *Corporate Fitness & Recreation, 4,* 26-29.

Guyton, A. (1974). *Function of the human body* (4th ed.). Philadelphia: W.B. Saunders.

Halcomb, R. (1983, October/November). Introducing a class act. *Corporate Fitness & Recreation,* 37-43.

Martens, R., Christina, R., Harvey, J., & Sharkey, B. (1981). *Coaching young athletes.* Champaign, IL: Human Kinetics.

Melleby, A. (1982). *The Y's way to a healthy back.* Piscataway, NJ: New Century.

Mirikin, G., & Hoffman, M. (1978). *The sportsmedicine book.* Boston: Little, Brown and Company.

Nygaard, G., & Boone, T. (1985). *Coaches guide to sport law.* Champaign, IL: Human Kinetics.

Richie, D.H., & Washington, E.L. (1983). Musculoskeletal problems in aerobic dancers—Part I. *Dance Medicine Health Newsletter, 2,* 9-11.

Rockefeller, K.A., & Burke, E.J. (1979). Psycho-physiological analysis of an aerobic dance programme for women. *British Journal of Physical Education*, **13**, 77-80.

Rogers, C. (1984). Books by exercise experts: Why aren't they working out? *The Physician and Sportsmedicine*, **12**, 143-150.

Scarantino, B. (1984, November/December). Get in step with choreography. *Aerobics & Fitness*, 28-30.

Southmayd, W., & Hoffman, M. (1981). *Sports Health*. New York: Quick Fox.

Strovas, J. (1984). Aerobic dance instructors are not injury proof. *The Physician and Sportsmedicine*, **12**, 24.

Town, G. (1985). *Science of triathlon training and competition*. Champaign, IL: Human Kinetics.

Vaccaro, P., & Clinton, M. (1981). The effects of aerobic dance conditioning on the body composition and maximal oxygen uptake of college women. *Journal of Sports Medicine and Physical Fitness*, **21**, 291-294.

Washington, E.L., Rosenberg, S.L., Friedlander, B., & Carlin, B. (1983). Musculoskeletal problems in aerobic dancers—Part II. *Dance Medicine Health Newsletter*, **2**, 11-12.

Weber, H. (1974). The energy cost of aerobic dancing. *Fitness for Living*, **8**, 26-30.

Wessel, J.A. (1970). *Movement fundamentals: Figure, form, fun* (3rd ed.). Englewood Cliffs, NJ: Prentice Hall.

Index

S

Safe exercises   56-67, 104
Safe workout environment   96-97, 105
Salary considerations   111
Selecting aerobic dance steps   48, 52
Self-confidence   98
Shin splints   78
Shock absorption   75
Shoes:
    general construction   85
    proper fit   86
Sport psychology   92
Sprains:
    Grade I   77
    Grade II   77
    Grade III   77
Stabilizers   57
Static stretching   24
Strains:
    Grade I   75
    Grade II   75
    Grade III   76
Stroke volume   12
Supine position   57

Systematic observation   51, 68-72
Systemic veins and arteries   10
Systolic pressure   13

T

Tapes   55
Teaching styles   98-100
Tendonitis   76
Treating injuries   87-88

V

Ventricles   10
Vocal cues   49

W

Waivers   108
Warming up   34
Warning signs   38
Water   84
Working out in cold weather—
    guidelines   46
Working out in hot weather—
    guidelines   45
Workout   36